SpringerBriefs in Statistics

For further volumes:
http://www.springer.com/series/8921

Ton J. Cleophas · Aeilko H. Zwinderman

Machine Learning in Medicine - Cookbook

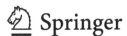 Springer

Ton J. Cleophas
Department Medicine
Albert Schweitzer Hospital
Sliedrecht
The Netherlands

Aeilko H. Zwinderman
Department Biostatistics and Epidemiology
Academic Medical Center
Amsterdam
The Netherlands

Additional material to this book can be downloaded from http://www.extras.springer.com.

ISSN 2191-544X   ISSN 2191-5458 (electronic)
ISBN 978-3-319-04180-3   ISBN 978-3-319-04181-0 (eBook)
DOI 10.1007/978-3-319-04181-0
Springer Cham Heidelberg New York Dordrecht London

Library of Congress Control Number: 2013957369

Printed on acid-free paper

Springer is part of Springer Science+Business Media (www.springer.com)

Preface

The amount of data stored in the world's databases doubles every 20 months, as estimated by Usama Fayyad, one of the founders of machine learning and coauthor of the book "Advances in knowledge discovery and data mining" (ed. by the American Association for Artificial Intelligence, Menlo Park, CA, USA, 1996), and clinicians, familiar with traditional statistical methods, are at a loss to analyze them.

Traditional methods have, indeed, difficulty to identify outliers in large datasets, and to find patterns in big data and data with multiple exposure/outcome variables. In addition, analysis rules for surveys and questionnaires, which are currently common methods of data collection, are, essentially, missing. Fortunately, the new discipline, machine learning, is able to cover all of these limitations.

In the past three years, we have completed three textbooks entitled "Machine Learning in Medicine Part One, Two, and Three" (ed. by Springer, Heidelberg, Germany, 2013). Although the textbooks were well received, it came to our attention that jaded physicians and students often lacked time to read the entire books, and requested a small book on the most important machine learning methods, without background information and theoretical discussions, and high-lighting technical details.

For this reason, we have produced a small cookbook of around 100 pages containing similar information as that of the textbooks, but in a condensed form. The chapters do not have "summary, introduction, discussion, and reference" sections. Only the "example and results" sections have been maintained. Physicians and students wishing more information are referred to the textbooks.

So far medical professionals have been rather reluctant to use machine learning.

Ravinda Khattree, coauthor of the book "Computational methods in biomedical research" (ed. by Chapman & Hall, Baton Rouge, LA, USA, 2007), suggests that there may be historical reasons: technological (doctors are better than computers (?)), legal, and cultural (doctors are better trusted). Also, in the field of diagnosis making, few doctors may want a computer checking them, are interested in collaboration with a computer, collaborate with computer engineers.

In the current book, we will demonstrate that machine learning performs sometimes better than traditional statistics does. For example, if the data perfectly fit the cut-offs for node splitting, because, e.g., age > 55 years gives an exponential rise in infarctions, then decision trees, optimal binning, and optimal scaling will be better analysis methods than traditional regression methods with age as continuous predictor. Machine learning may have little options for adjusting confounding and interaction, but you can add propensity scores and interaction variables to almost any machine learning method.

Twenty machine leaning methods relevant to medicine are described. Each chapter starts with purposes and scientific questions. Then, step-by-step analyses, using mostly simulated data examples, are given. In order for readers to perform their own analyses, the data examples are available at extras.springer.com. Finally, a paragraph with conclusion, and reference to the corresponding sites of the three textbooks written by the same authors, is given. We should emphasize that all of the methods described have been successfully applied in the authors' own research.

Lyon, November 2013   Ton J. Cleophas
                                                                   Aeilko H. Zwinderman

Contents

Part III Rules Models

Part I
Cluster Models

Chapter 1
Hierarchical Clustering and K-means Clustering to Identify Subgroups in Surveys (50 Patients)

General Purpose

Clusters are subgroups in a survey estimated by the distances between the values needed to connect the patients, otherwise called cases. It is an important methodology in explorative data mining.

Specific Scientific Question

In a survey of patients with mental depression of different ages and depression scores, how do different clustering methods perform in identifying so far unobserved subgroups.

1	2	3
20.00	8.00	1
21.00	7.00	2
23.00	9.00	3
24.00	10.00	4
25.00	8.00	5
26.00	9.00	6
27.00	7.00	7
28.00	8.00	8
24.00	9.00	9
32.00	9.00	10
30.00	1.00	11
40.00	2.00	12

(continued)

T. J. Cleophas and A. H. Zwinderman, *Machine Learning in Medicine - Cookbook*,
SpringerBriefs in Statistics, DOI: 10.1007/978-3-319-04181-0_1,
© The Author(s) 2014

In the output a dendrogram of the results is given. The actual distances between the cases are rescaled to fall into a range of 0–25 units (0 = minimal distance, 25 = maximal distance). The cases no. 1–11, 21–25 are clustered together in cluster 1, the cases 12, 13, 20, 26, 27, 31, 32, 35, 40 in cluster 2, both at a rescaled distance from 0 at approximately 3 units, the remainder of the cases is clustered at approximately 6 units. And so, as requested, three clusters have been indentified with cases more similar to one another than to the other clusters. When minimizing the output, the data file comes up and it now shows the cluster membership of each case. We will use SPSS again to draw a Dotter graph of the data.

Command:
Analyze....Graphs....Legacy Dialogs: click Simple Scatter....Define....Y-axis: enter Depression Score....X-axis: enter Age....OK.

The graph (with age on the x-axis and severity score on the y-axis) produced by SPSS shows the cases. Using Microsoft's drawing commands we can encircle the clusters as identified. All of them are oval and even, approximately, round, because variables have similar scales, but they are different in size.

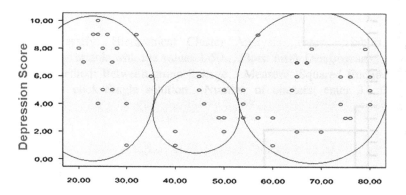

K-means Cluster Analysis

Command:
Analyze....Classify....K-means Cluster Analysis....Variables: enter Age and Depression score....Label Cases by: patient number as a string variable....Number of clusters: 3 (in our example chosen for comparison with the above method)....click Method: mark Iterate....click Iterate: Maximal Iterations: mark 10....Convergence criterion: mark 0....click Continue....click Save: mark Cluster Membership....click Continue....click Options: mark Initiate cluster centers....mark ANOVA table.... mark Cluster information for each case....click Continue....OK.

The output shows that the three clusters identified by the k-means cluster model were significantly different from one another both by testing the y-axis (depression score) and the x-axis variable (age). When minimizing the output sheets, the data file comes up and shows the cluster membership of the three clusters.

ANOVA						
	Cluster		Error		F	Sig.
	Mean square	df	Mean square	df		
Age	8712.723	2	31.082	47	280.310	0.000
Depression score	39.102	2	4.593	47	8.513	0.001

We will use SPSS again to draw a Dotter graph of the data.

Command:
Analyze....Graphs....Legacy Dialogs: click Simple Scatter....Define....Y-axis: enter Depression Score....X-axis: enter Age....OK.

The graph (with age on the x-axis and severity score on the y-axis) produced by SPSS shows the cases. Using Microsoft's drawing commands we can encircle the clusters as identified. All of them are oval and even approximately round because variables have similar scales, and they are approximately equal in size.

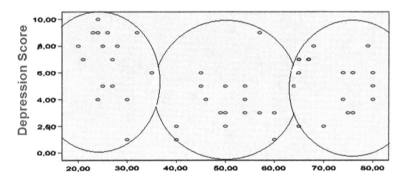

Conclusion

Clusters are estimated by the distances between the values needed to connect the cases. It is an important methodology in explorative data mining. Hierarchical clustering is adequate if subgroups are expected to be different in size, k-means Clustering if approximately similar in size. Density-based clustering is more appropriate if small outlier groups between otherwise homogenous populations are expected. The latter method is in Chap. 2.

Note

More background, theoretical and mathematical information of the two methods is given in Machine Learning in Medicine Part Two, Chap. 8 Two-dimensional Clustering, pp. 65–75, Springer Heidelberg Germany 2013. Density-based clustering will be reviewed in the next chapter.

Chapter 2
Density-Based Clustering to Identify Outlier Groups in Otherwise Homogeneous Data (50 Patients)

General Purpose

Clusters are subgroups in a survey estimated by the distances between the values needed to connect the patients, otherwise called cases. It is an important methodology in explorative data mining. Density-based clustering is used.

Specific Scientific Question

In a survey of patients with mental depression of different ages and depression scores, how does density-based clustering perform in identifying so far unobserved subgroups.

1	2	3
20.00	8.00	1
21.00	7.00	2
23.00	9.00	3
24.00	10.00	4
25.00	8.00	5
26.00	9.00	6
27.00	7.00	7
28.00	8.00	8
24.00	9.00	9
32.00	9.00	10
30.00	1.00	11
40.00	2.00	12
50.00	3.00	13
60.00	1.00	14
70.00	2.00	15
76.00	3.00	16

(continued)

T. J. Cleophas and A. H. Zwinderman, *Machine Learning in Medicine - Cookbook*, SpringerBriefs in Statistics, DOI: 10.1007/978-3-319-04181-0_2, © The Author(s) 2014

(continued)

1	2	3
65.00	2.00	17
54.00	3.00	18

Var 1 age
Var 2 depression score (0 = very mild, 10 = severest)
Var 3 patient number (called cases here)
Only the first 18 patients are given, the entire data file is entitled
"hierk-meansdensity" and is in extras.springer.com.

Density-Based Cluster Analysis

The DBSCAN method was used (density based spatial clustering of application
with noise). As this method is not available in SPSS, an interactive JAVA Applet
freely available at the Internet was used [Data Clustering Applets. http://
webdocs.cs.ualberts.ca/ ~ yaling/Cluster/applet]. The DBSCAN connects points
that satisfy a density criterion given by a minimum number of patients within a
defined radius (radius = Eps; minimum number = Min pts).

Command:
User Define....Choose data set: remove values given....enter you own x and y
values....Choose algorithm: select DBSCAN....Eps: mark 25....Min pts: mark
3....Start....Show.

Three cluster memberships are again shown. We will use SPSS 19.0 again to
draw a Dotter graph of the data.

Command:
Analyze....Graphs....Legacy Dialogs: click Simple Scatter....Define....Y-axis:
enter Depression Score....X-axis: enter Age....OK.

The graph (with age on the x-axis and severity score on the y-axis) shows the
cases. Using Microsoft's drawing commands we can encircle the clusters as
identified. Two very small ones, one large one. All of the clusters identified are
non-circular and, are, obviously, based on differences in patient-density.

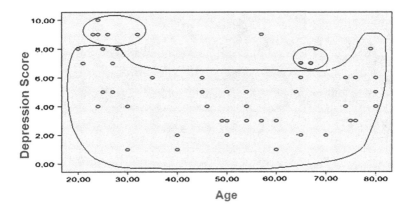

Conclusion

Clusters are estimated by the distances between the values needed to connect the cases. It is an important methodology in explorative data mining. Density-based clustering is suitable if small outlier groups between otherwise homogeneous populations are expected. Hierarchical and k-means clustering are more appropriate if subgroups have Gaussian-like patterns (Chap. 1).

Note

More background, theoretical and mathematical information of the three methods is given in Machine Learning in Medicine Part Two, Chap. 8. Two-dimensional Clustering, pp. 65–75, Springer Heidelberg Germany 2013. Hierarchical and k-means clustering are reviewed in the previous chapter.

Chapter 3
Two Step Clustering to Identify Subgroups and Predict Subgroup Memberships in Individual Future Patients (120 Patients)

General Purpose

To assess whether two step clustering of survey data can be trained to identify subgroups and subgroup membership.

Specific Scientific Question

In patients with mental depression, can the item scores of depression severity be used to classify subgroups and to predict subgroup membership of future patients.

Var 1	Var 2	Var 3	Var 4	Var 5	Var 6	Var 7	Var 8	Var 9
9.00	9.00	9.00	2.00	2.00	2.00	2.00	2.00	2.00
8.00	8.00	6.00	3.00	3.00	3.00	3.00	3.00	3.00
7.00	7.00	7.00	4.00	4.00	4.00	4.00	4.00	4.00
4.00	9.00	9.00	2.00	2.00	6.00	2.00	2.00	2.00
8.00	8.00	8.00	3.00	3.00	3.00	3.00	3.00	3.00
7.00	7.00	7.00	4.00	4.00	4.00	4.00	4.00	4.00
9.00	5.00	9.00	9.00	2.00	2.00	2.00	2.00	2.00
8.00	8.00	8.00	3.00	3.00	3.00	3.00	3.00	3.00
7.00	7.00	7.00	4.00	6.00	4.00	4.00	4.00	4.00
9.00	9.00	9.00	2.00	2.00	2.00	2.00	2.00	2.00
4.00	4.00	4.00	9.00	9.00	9.00	3.00	3.00	3.00
3.00	3.00	3.00	8.00	8.00	8.00	4.00	4.00	4.00

Var 1–9 = depression score 1–9

Only the first 12 patients are given, the entire data file is entitled "twostep-clustering" and is in extras.springer.com.

T. J. Cleophas and A. H. Zwinderman, *Machine Learning in Medicine - Cookbook*, SpringerBriefs in Statistics, DOI: 10.1007/978-3-319-04181-0_3, © The Author(s) 2014

The Computer Teaches Itself to Make Predictions

SPSS 19.0 is used for data analysis. It will use XML (eXtended Markup Language) files to store data. Now start by opening the data file.

Command:
Click Transform....click Random Number Generators....click Set Starting Point ....click Fixed Value (2000000)....click OK....click Analyze....Classify....Two-Step Cluster....Continuous Variables: enter depression 1–9....click Output: in Working Data File click Create cluster membership....in XML Files click Export final model....click Browse....File name: enter "export2step"....click Save....click Continue....click OK.

Returning to the data file we will observe that 3 subgroups have been identified and for each patient the subgroup membership is given as a novel variable, and the name of this novel variable is TSC (two step cluster). The saved XML file will now be used to compute the predicted subgroup membership in five future patients. For convenience the XML file is given in extras.springer.com.

Var 1	Var 2	Var 3	Var 4	Var 5	Var 6	Var 7	Var 8	Var 9
4.00	5.00	3.00	4.00	6.00	9.00	8.00	7.00	6.00
2.00	2.00	2.00	2.00	2.00	2.00	2.00	2.00	2.00
5.00	4.00	6.00	7.00	6.00	5.00	3.00	4.00	5.00
9.00	8.00	7.00	6.00	5.00	4.00	3.00	2.00	2.00
7.00	7.00	7.00	3.00	3.00	3.00	9.00	9.00	9.00

Var 1–9 = Depression score 1–9

Enter the above data in a new SPSS data file.

Command:
Utilities....click Scoring Wizard....click Browse....click Select....Folder: enter the export2step.xml file....click Select....in Scoring Wizard click Next....click Use value substitution....click Next....click Finish.

The above data file now gives subgroup memberships of the 5 patients as computed by the two step cluster model with the help of the XML file.

Var 1	Var 2	Var 3	Var 4	Var 5	Var 6	Var 7	Var 8	Var 9	Var 10
4.00	5.00	3.00	4.00	6.00	9.00	8.00	7.00	6.00	2.00
2.00	2.00	2.00	2.00	2.00	2.00	2.00	2.00	2.00	2.00
5.00	4.00	6.00	7.00	6.00	5.00	3.00	4.00	5.00	3.00
9.00	8.00	7.00	6.00	5.00	4.00	3.00	2.00	2.00	1.00
7.00	7.00	7.00	3.00	3.00	3.00	9.00	9.00	9.00	2.00

Var 1–9 = Depression score 1–9
Var 10 = predicted value

Conclusion

Two step clustering can be readily trained to identify subgroups in patients with mental depression, and, with the help of an XML file, it can, subsequently, be used to identify subgroup memberships in individual future patients.

Note

More background, theoretical and mathematical information of two step and other methods of clustering is available in Machine Learning Part Two, Chaps. 8 and 9, entitled "Two-dimensional clustering" and "Multidimensional clustering", pp. 65–75 and 77–91, Springer Heidelberg Germany 2013.

Part II
Linear Models

Chapter 4
Linear, Logistic, and Cox Regression for Outcome Prediction with Unpaired Data (20, 55, and 60 Patients)

General Purpose

To assess whether linear, logistic and Cox modeling can be used to train clinical data samples to make predictions about groups and individual patients.

Specific Scientific Question

How many hours will patients sleep, how large is the risk for patients to fall out of bed, how large is the hazard for patients to die.

Linear Regression, the Computer Teaches Itself to Make Predictions

Var 1	Var 2	Var 3	Var 4	Var 5
0.00	6.00	65.00	0.00	1.00
0.00	7.10	75.00	0.00	1.00
0.00	8.10	86.00	0.00	0.00
0.00	7.50	74.00	0.00	0.00
0.00	6.40	64.00	0.00	1.00
0.00	7.90	75.00	1.00	1.00
0.00	6.80	65.00	1.00	1.00
0.00	6.60	64.00	1.00	0.00
0.00	7.30	75.00	1.00	0.00
0.00	5.60	56.00	0.00	0.00
1.00	5.10	55.00	1.00	0.00
1.00	8.00	85.00	0.00	1.00

(continued)

T. J. Cleophas and A. H. Zwinderman, *Machine Learning in Medicine - Cookbook*, SpringerBriefs in Statistics, DOI: 10.1007/978-3-319-04181-0_4, © The Author(s) 2014

(continued)

Var 1	Var 2	Var 3	Var 4	Var 5
1.00	3.80	36.00	1.00	0.00
1.00	4.40	47.00	0.00	1.00
1.00	5.20	58.00	1.00	0.00
1.00	5.40	56.00	0.00	1.00
1.00	4.30	46.00	1.00	1.00
1.00	6.00	64.00	1.00	0.00
1.00	3.70	33.00	1.00	0.00
1.00	6.20	65.00	0.00	1.00

Var 1 = treatment 0 is placebo, treatment 1 is sleeping pill
Var 2 = hours of sleep
Var 3 = age
Var 4 = gender
Var 5 = comorbidity

SPSS 19.0 is used for analysis, with the help of an eXtended Markup Language (XML) file. The data file is entitled "linoutcomeprediction" and is in extras. springer.com. Start by opening the data file.

Command:
Click Transform....click Random Number Generators....click Set Starting Point ....click Fixed Value (2000000)....click OK....click Analyze....Regression.... Linear....Dependent: enter hoursofsleep....Independent: enter treatment and age....click Save....Predicted Values: click Unstandardized....in XML Files click Export final model....click Browse....File name: enter "exportlin"....click Save....click Continue....click OK.

Coefficients[a]

Model		Unstandardized coefficients		Standardized coefficients	t	Sig.
		B	Std. error	Beta		
1.	(Constant)	0.989	0.366		2.702	0.015
	Treatment	−0.411	0.143	−0.154	−2.878	0.010
	Age	0.085	0.005	0.890	16.684	0.000

[a] Dependent Variable: hours of sleep

The output sheets show in the coefficients table that both treatment and age are significant predictors at $p < 0.10$. Returning to the data file we will observe that SPSS has computed predicted values and gives them in a novel variable entitled PRE_1. The saved XML file will now be used to compute the predicted hours of sleep in 4 novel patients with the following characteristics. For convenience the XML file is given in extras.springer.com.

Var 1	Var 2	Var 3	Var 4	Var 5
0.00	6.00	66.00	0.00	1.00
0.00	7.10	74.00	0.00	1.00
0.00	8.10	86.00	0.00	0.00
0.00	7.50	74.00	0.00	0.00

Var 1 = treatment 0 is placebo, treatment 1 is sleeping pill
Var 2 = hours of sleep
Var 3 = age
Var 4 = gender
Var 5 = comorbidity

Enter the above data in a new SPSS data file.

Command:
Utilities....click Scoring Wizard....click Browse....click Select....Folder: enter the exportlin.xml file....click Select....in Scoring Wizard click Next....click Use value substitution....click Next....click Finish.

The above data file now gives individually predicted hours of sleep as computed by the linear model with the help of the XML file.

Var 1	Var 2	Var 3	Var 4	Var 5	Var 6
0.00	6.00	66.00	0.00	1.00	6.51
0.00	7.10	74.00	0.00	1.00	7.28
0.00	8.10	86.00	0.00	0.00	8.30
0.00	7.50	74.00	0.00	0.00	7.28

Var 1 = treatment 0 is placebo, treatment 1 is sleeping pill
Var 2 = hours of sleep
Var 3 = age
Var 4 = gender
Var 5 = comorbidity
Var 6 = predicted hours of sleep

Conclusion

The module linear regression can be readily trained to predict hours of sleep both in groups and, with the help of an XML file, in individual future patients.

Note

More background, theoretical and mathematical information of linear regression is available in Statistics Applied to Clinical Studies, 5th Ed, Chaps. 14 and 15, entitled "Linear regression basic approach" and "Linear regression for assessing precision, confounding, interaction", pp. 161–176 and 177–185, Springer Heidelberg Germany 2012.

Logistic Regression, the Computer Teaches Itself to Make Predictions

Var 1	Var 2	Var 3	Var 4	Var 5
0.00	1.00	50.00	0.00	1.00
0.00	1.00	76.00	0.00	1.00
0.00	1.00	57.00	1.00	1.00
0.00	1.00	65.00	0.00	1.00
0.00	1.00	46.00	1.00	1.00
0.00	1.00	36.00	1.00	1.00
0.00	1.00	98.00	0.00	0.00
0.00	1.00	56.00	1.00	0.00
0.00	1.00	44.00	0.00	0.00
0.00	1.00	76.00	1.00	1.00
0.00	1.00	75.00	1.00	1.00
0.00	1.00	74.00	1.00	1.00
0.00	1.00	87.00	0.00	0.00

Var 1 = department type
Var 2 = falling out of bed (1 = yes)
Var 3 = age
Var 4 = gender
Var 5 = letter of complaint (1 = yes)

Only the first 13 patients are given, the entire data file is entitled "logout-comeprediction" and is in extras.springer.com.

SPSS 19.0 is used for analysis, with the help of an eXtended Markup Language (XML) file. Start by opening the data file.

Command:
Click Transform....click Random Number Generators....click Set Starting Point ....click Fixed Value (2000000)....click OK....click Analyze....Regression ....Binary Logistic....Dependent: enter fallingoutofbed ....Covariates: enter departmenttype and letterofcomplaint....click Save....in Predicted Values click Probabilities....in Export model information to XML file click Browse.... File name: enter "exportlog"....click Save....click Continue....click OK.

Variables in the equation		B	S.E.	Wald	df	Sig.	Exp(B)
Step 1[a]	Department type	1.349	0.681	3.930	1	0.047	3.854
	Letter of complaint	2.039	0.687	8.816	1	0.003	7.681
	Constant	−1.007	0.448	5.047	1	0.025	0.365

[a] Variable(s) entered on step 1: department type, letter of complaint

In the above output table it is shown that both department type and letter of complaint are significant predictors of the risk of falling out of bed. Returning to the data file we will observe that SPSS has computed predicted values and gives them in a novel variable entitled PRE_1. The saved XML file will now be used to compute the predicted probability of falling out of bed in 5 novel patients with the following characteristics. For convenience the XML file is given in extras.springer.com.

Var 1	Var 2	Var 3	Var 4	Var 5
0.00		67.00	0.00	0.00
1.00		54.00	1.00	0.00
1.00		65.00	1.00	0.00
1.00		74.00	1.00	1.00
1.00		73.00	0.00	1.00

Var 1 = department type
Var 2 = falling out of bed (1 = yes)
Var 3 = age
Var 4 = gender
Var 5 = letter of complaint (1 = yes)

Enter the above data in a new SPSS data file.

Command:
Utilities....click Scoring Wizard....click Browse....click Select....Folder: enter the exportlog.xml file....click Select....in Scoring Wizard click Next....mark Probability of Predicted Category....click Next....click Finish.

The above data file now gives individually predicted probabilities of falling out of bed as computed by the logistic model with the help of the XML file.

Var 1	Var 2	Var 3	Var 4	Var 5	Var 6
0.00		67.00	0.00	0.00	0.73
1.00		54.00	1.00	0.00	0.58
1.00		65.00	1.00	0.00	0.58
1.00		74.00	1.00	1.00	0.92
1.00		73.00	0.00	1.00	0.92

Var 1 = department type
Var 2 = falling out of bed (1 = yes)
Var 3 = age
Var 4 = gender
Var 5 = letter of complaint (1 = yes)
Var 6 = predicted probability

Conclusion

The module binary logistic regression can be readily trained to predict probability of falling out of bed both in groups and, with the help of an XML file, in individual future patients.

Note

More background, theoretical and mathematical information of binary logistic regression is available in Statistics Applied to Clinical Studies, 5th Ed, Chaps. 17, 19, and 65, entitled "Logistic and , Markov models, Laplace transformations", "Post-hoc analyses in clinical trials", and "Odds ratios and multiple regression", pp. 199–218, 227–231, and 695–711, Springer Heidelberg Germany 2012.

Cox Regression, the Computer Teaches Itself to Make Predictions

Var 1	Var 2	Var 3	Var 4
1.00	1.00	0.00	65.00
1.00	1.00	0.00	66.00
2.00	1.00	0.00	73.00
2.00	1.00	0.00	91.00
2.00	1.00	0.00	86.00
2.00	1.00	0.00	87.00
2.00	1.00	0.00	54.00
2.00	1.00	0.00	66.00
2.00	1.00	0.00	64.00
3.00	0.00	0.00	62.00
4.00	1.00	0.00	57.00
5.00	1.00	0.00	85.00
6.00	1.00	0.00	85.00

Var 1 = follow up in months
Var 2 = event (1 = yes)
Var 3 = treatment modality
Var 4 = age

Only the first 13 patients are given, the entire data file is entitled "Coxoutcomeprediction" and is in extras.springer.com.

SPSS 19.0 is used for analysis, with the help of an XML (eXtended Markup Language) file. Start by opening the data file.

Command:
Click Transform....click Random Number Generators....click Set Starting Point
....click Fixed Value (2000000)....click OK....click Analyze....Survival....Cox
Regression....Time: followupmonth....Status: event....Define event: enter 1....
Covariates: enter treatment and age....click Save....mark: Survival function.... In
Export Model information to XML file click Browse.... File name: enter
"exportCox"....click Save....click Continue....click OK.

Variables in the Equation						
	B	SE	Wald	df	Sig.	Exp(B)
Treatment	−0.791	0.332	5.686	1	0.017	0.454
age	0.028	0.012	5.449	1	0.020	1.028

In the above output table it is shown that both treatment modality and age are
significant predictors of survival. Returning to the data file we will now observe
that SPSS has computed individual probabilities of survival and gave them in a
novel variable entitled SUR_1. The probabilities vary from 0.00 to 1.00. E.g., for
the first patient, based on follow up of 1 month, treatment modality 0, and age 65,
the computer has computed a mean survival chance at the time of observation of
0.95741 (= over 95 %). Other patients had much less probability of survival. If
you would have limited sources for further treatment in this population, it would
make sense not to burden with continued treatment those with, e.g., less than 20 %
survival probability. We should emphasize that the probability is based on the
information of the variables 1, 3, 4, and is assumed to be measured just prior to the
event, and the event is not taken into account here.

Var 1	Var 2	Var 3	Var 4	SUR_1
1.00	1.00	0.00	65.00	0.95741

The saved XML file will now be used to compute the predicted probabilities of
survival in 5 novel patients with the following characteristics. For convenience the
XML file is given in extras.springer.com. We will skip the variable 2 for the above
reason.

Var 1	Var 2	Var 3	Var 4
30.00		1.00	88.00
29.00		1.00	67.00
29.00		1.00	56.00
29.00		1.00	54.00

(continued)

(continued)

Var 1	Var 2	Var 3	Var 4
28.00		1.00	57.00

Var 1 = follow up in months
Var 2 = event (1 = yes)
Var 3 = treatment modality
Var 4 = age

Enter the above data in a new SPSS data file.

Command:
Utilities....click Scoring Wizard....click Browse....click Select....Folder: enter the exportCox.xml file....click Select....in Scoring Wizard click Next....mark Predicted Value....click Next....click Finish.

The above data file now gives individually predicted probabilities of survival as computed by the Cox regression model with the help of the XML file.

Var 1	Var 2	Var 3	Var 4	Var 5 Predicted Value
30.00		1.00	88.00	0.18
29.00		1.00	67.00	0.39
29.00		1.00	56.00	0.50
29.00		1.00	54.00	0.51
28.00		1.00	57.00	0.54

Var 1 = follow up in months
Var 2 = event (1 = yes)
Var 3 = treatment modality
Var 4 = age
Var 5 = predicted probability of survival (0.0–1.0)

Conclusion

The module Cox regression can be readily trained to predict probability of survival both in groups and, with the help of an XML file, in individual future patients. Like with linear and logistic regression models, Cox regression is an important method to determine with limited health care sources, who of the patients will be recommended expensive medications and other treatments.

Note

More background, theoretical and mathematical information of binary logistic regression is available in Statistics Applied to Clinical Studies, 5th Ed, Chaps. 17

and 31, entitled "Logistic and Cox regression, Markov models, Laplace transformations", and "Time-dependent factor analysis", pp. 199–218, and pp. 353–364, Springer Heidelberg Germany 2012.

Chapter 5
Generalized Linear Models for Outcome Prediction with Paired Data (100 Patients and 139 Physicians)

General Purpose

With linear and logistic regression *unpaired* data can be used for outcome prediction. With generalized linear models *paired* data can be used for the purpose.

Specific Scientific Question

Can crossover studies (1) of sleeping pills and (2) of lifestyle treatments be used as training samples to predict hours of sleep and lifestyle treatment in groups and individuals.

Generalized Linear Modeling, the Computer Teaches Itself to Make Predictions

Var 1	Var 2	Var 3	Var 4
6.10	79.00	1.00	1.00
5.20	79.00	1.00	2.00
7.00	55.00	2.00	1.00
7.90	55.00	2.00	2.00
8.20	78.00	3.00	1.00
3.90	78.00	3.00	2.00
7.60	53.00	4.00	1.00
4.70	53.00	4.00	2.00
6.50	85.00	5.00	1.00
5.30	85.00	5.00	2.00

(continued)

T. J. Cleophas and A. H. Zwinderman, *Machine Learning in Medicine - Cookbook*, SpringerBriefs in Statistics, DOI: 10.1007/978-3-319-04181-0_5, © The Author(s) 2014

(continued)

Var 1	Var 2	Var 3	Var 4
8.40	85.00	6.00	1.00
5.40	85.00	6.00	2.00

Var 1 = outcome (hours of sleep after sleeping pill or placebo)
Var 2 = age
Var 3 = patient number (patient id)
Var 4 = treatment modality (1 sleeping pill, 2 placebo)

Only the data from first 6 patients are given, the entire data file is entitled "generalizedlmpairedcontinuous" and is in extras.springer.com. SPSS 19.0 is used for analysis, with the help of an XML (eXtended Markup Language) file. Start by opening the data file.

Command:
Click Transform....click Random Number Generators....click Set Starting Point ....click Fixed Value (2000000)....click OK....click Analyze....Generalized Linear Models....again click Generalized Linear models....click Type of Model....click Linear....click Response....Dependent Variable: enter Outcome....Scale Weight Variable: enter patientid....click Predictors....Factors: enter treatment.... Covariates: enter age....click Model: Model: enter treatment and age....click Save: mark Predicted value of linear predictor....click Export....click Browse....File name: enter "exportpairedcontinuous"....click Save....click Continue....click OK.

Parameter estimates

Parameter	B	Stri. error	95 % Wald confidence interval		Hypothesis test		
			Lower	Upper	Wald Chi-square	df	Sig.
(Intercept)	6.178	0.5171	5.165	7.191	142.763	1	0.000
[Treatments = 0.00]	2.003	0.2089	1.593	2.412	91.895	1	0.000
[Treatment = 2,00]	0[a]						
Age	−0.014	0.0075	−0.029	0.001	3.418	1	0.064
(Scale)	27.825[b]	3.9351	21.089	36.713			

Dependent variable: outcome
Model: (Intercept), treatment, age
[a] Set to zero because this parameter is redundant
[b] Maximum likelihood estimate

The output sheets show that both treatment and age are significant predictors at $p < 0.10$. Returning to the data file we will observe that SPSS has computed predicted values of hours of sleep, and has given them in a novel variable entitled XBPredicted (predicted values of linear predictor). The saved XML file entitled "exportpairedcontinuous" will now be used to compute the predicted hours of sleep in five novel patients with the following characteristics. For convenience the XML file is given in extras.springer.com.

Var 2	Var 3	Var 4
79.00	1.00	1.00
55.00	2.00	1.00
78.00	3.00	1.00
53.00	4.00	2.00
85.00	5.00	1.00

Var 2 = age
Var 3 = patient number (patient id)
Var 4 = treatment modality (1 sleeping pill, 2 placebo)

Enter the above data in a new SPSS data file.

Command:
Utilities....click Scoring Wizard....click Browse....click Select....Folder: enter the exportpairedcontinuous.xml file....click Select....in Scoring Wizard click Next....click Use value substitution....click Next....click Finish.

The above data file now gives individually predicted hours of sleep as computed by the linear model with the help of the XML file.

Var 2	Var 3	Var 4	Var 5
79.00	1.00	1.00	7.09
55.00	2.00	1.00	7.42
78.00	3.00	1.00	7.10
53.00	4.00	2.00	5.44
85.00	5.00	1.00	7.00

Var 2 = age
Var 3 = patient number (patient id)
Var 4 = treatment modality (1 sleeping pill, 2 placebo)
Var 5 = predicted values of hours of sleep in individual patient

Conclusion

The module generalized linear models can be readily trained to predict hours of sleep in groups, and, with the help of an XML file, in individual future patients.

Generalized Estimation Equations, the Computer Teaches Itself to Make Predictions

Var 1	Var 2	Var 3	Var 4
0.00	89.00	1.00	1.00
0.00	89.00	1.00	2.00
0.00	78.00	2.00	1.00
0.00	78.00	2.00	2.00
0.00	79.00	3.00	1.00
0.00	79.00	3.00	2.00
0.00	76.00	4.00	1.00
0.00	76.00	4.00	2.00
0.00	87.00	5.00	1.00
0.00	87.00	5.00	2.00
0.00	84.00	6.00	1.00
0.00	84.00	6.00	2.00
0.00	84.00	7.00	1.00
0.00	84.00	7.00	2.00
0.00	69.00	8.00	1.00
0.00	69.00	8.00	2.00
0.00	77.00	9.00	1.00
0.00	77.00	9.00	2.00
0.00	79.00	10.00	1.00
0.00	79.00	10.00	2.00

Var 1 = outcome (lifestyle advise given 0 = no, 1 = yes)
Var 2 = physicians' age
Var 3 = physicians' id
Var 4 = prior postgraduate education regarding lifestyle advise (1= no, 2 = sssyes)

Only the first 10 physicians are given, the entire data file is entitled "generalizedpairedbinary" and is in extras.springer.com. All physicians are assessed twice, once before lifestyle education and once after. The effect of lifestyle education on the willingness to provide lifestyle advise was the main objective of the study.

SPSS 19.0 is used for analysis, with the help of an XML (eXtended Markup Language) file. Start by opening the data file.

Command:
Click Transform....click Random Number Generators....click Set Starting Point ....click Fixed Value (2000000)....click OK....click Analyze....Generalized Linear Models....Generalized Estimating Equations....click Repeated....in Subjects variables enter physicianid....in Within-subject variables enter lifestyle advise....in Structure enter Unstructured....click Type of Model....mark Binary logistic....click Response....in Dependent Variable enter outcome....click

Reference Category....mark First....click Continue....click Predictors....in Factors enter lifestyleadvise....in Covariates enter age....click Model....in Model enter lifestyle and age....click Save....mark Predicted value of mean of response....click Export....mark Export model in XML....click Browse.... In File name: enter "exportpairedbinary"....in Look in: enter the appropriate map in your computer for storage....click Save....click Continue....click OK.

Parameter estimates

Parameter	B	Std. Error	95 % Wald confidence interval		Hypothesis test		
			Lower	Upper	Wald Chi-square	df	Sig.
(Intercept)	2.469	0.7936	0.913	4.024	9.677	1	0.002
Lifestyleadvise = 1,00]	−0.522	0.2026	−0.919	−0.124	6.624	1	0.010
Lifestyleadvise = 2,00]	0[a]						
Age	−0.042	0.0130	−0.068	−0.017	10.563	1	0.001
(Scale)	1						

Dependent variable: outcome
Model: (Intercept), lifestyleadvise, age
[a] Set to zero because this parameter is redundant

The output sheets show that both prior lifestyle education and physicians' age are very significant predictors at $p < 0.01$. Returning to the data file we will observe that SPSS has computed predicted probabilities of lifestyle advise given or not by each physician in the data file, and a novel variable is added to the data file for the purpose. It is given the name MeanPredicted. The saved XML file entitled "exportpairedbinary" will now be used to compute the predicted probability of receiving lifestyle advise based on physicians' age and the physicians' prior lifestyle education in twelve novel physicians. For convenience the XML file is given in extras.springer.com.

Var 2	Var 3	Var 4
64.00	1.00	2.00
64.00	2.00	1.00
65.00	3.00	1.00
65.00	3.00	2.00
52.00	4.00	1.00
66.00	5.00	1.00
79.00	6.00	1.00
79.00	6.00	2.00
53.00	7.00	1.00
53.00	7.00	2.00

(continued)

(continued)

Var 2	Var 3	Var 4
55.00	8.00	1.00
46.00	9.00	1.00

Var 2 = age
Var 3 = physicianid
Var 4 = lifestyleadvise [prior postgraduate education regarding lifestyle advise (1 = no, 2 = yes)]

Enter the above data in a new SPSS data file.

Command:
Utilities....click Scoring Wizard....click Browse....click Select....Folder: enter the exportpairedbinary.xml file....click Select....in Scoring Wizard click Next....mark Probability of Predicted Category....click Next....click Finish.

The above data file now gives individually predicted probabilities of physicians giving lifestyle advise as computed by the logistic model with the help of the XML file.

Var 2	Var 3	Var 4	Var 5
64.00	1.00	2.00	0.56
64.00	2.00	1.00	0.68
65.00	3.00	1.00	0.69
65.00	3.00	2.00	0.57
52.00	4.00	1.00	0.56
66.00	5.00	1.00	0.70
79.00	6.00	1.00	0.80
79.00	6.00	2.00	0.70
53.00	7.00	1.00	0.57
53.00	7.00	2.00	0.56
55.00	8.00	1.00	0.59
46.00	9.00	1.00	0.50

Var 2 = age
Var 3 = physicianid
Var 4 = lifestyleadvise
Var 5 = probability of physicians giving lifestyle advise (between 0.0 and 1.0)

Conclusion

The module generalized estimating equations can be readily trained to predict with paired data the probability of physicians giving lifestyle advise as groups and, with the help of an XML file, as individual physicians.

Note

More background, theoretical and mathematical information of paired analysis of binary data is given in SPSS for Starters Part Two, Chap. 13, entitled "Paired binary (McNemar test)", pp. 47–49, Springer Heidelberg, Germany, 2010.

Chapter 6
Generalized Linear Models for Predicting Event-Rates (50 Patients)

General Purpose

To assess whether in a longitudinal study event rates, defined as numbers of events per person per period, can be analyzed with the generalized linear model module.

Specific Scientific Question

Can generalized linear modeling be trained to predict rates of episodes of paroxysmal atrial fibrillation both in groups and in individual future patients.

Fifty patients were followed for numbers of episodes of paroxysmal atrial fibrillation (PAF), while on treatment with two parallel treatment modalities. The data file is below.

Var 1	Var 2	Var 3	Var 4	Var 5
1	56.99	42.45	73	4
1	37.09	46.82	73	4
0	32.28	43.57	76	2
0	29.06	43.57	74	3
0	6.75	27.25	73	3
0	61.65	48.41	62	13
0	56.99	40.74	66	11
1	10.39	15.36	72	7
1	50.53	52.12	63	10
1	49.47	42.45	68	9
0	39.56	36.45	72	4
1	33.74	13.13	74	5

Var 1 = treatment modality
Var 2 = psychological score
Var 3 = social score
Var 4 = days of observation
Var 5 = number of episodes of paroxysmal atrial fibrillation (PAF) per day

T. J. Cleophas and A. H. Zwinderman, *Machine Learning in Medicine - Cookbook*, SpringerBriefs in Statistics, DOI: 10.1007/978-3-319-04181-0_6, © The Author(s) 2014

The first 12 patients are shown only, the entire data file is entitled "generalizedlmeventrates" and is in extras.springer.com.

The Computer Teaches Itself to Make Predictions

SPSS 19.0 is used for training and outcome prediction. It uses eXtended Markup Language (XML) files to store data. We will perform the analysis with a linear regression analysis of variable 5 as outcome variable and the other 4 variables as predictors. Start by opening the data file.

Command:
Analyze....Regression....Linear....Dependent Variable: episodes of paroxysmal atrial fibrillation....Independent: treatment modality, psychological score, social score, days of observation....OK.

Model		Coefficients[a]			t	Sig.
		Unstandardized coefficients		Standardized coefficients		
		B	Std. error	Beta		
1	(Constant)	49.059	5.447		9.006	0.000
	treat	−2.914	1.385	−0.204	−2.105	0.041
	psych	0.014	0.052	0.036	−0.273	0.786
	soc	−0.073	0.058	−0.169	−1.266	0.212
	days	−0.557	0.074	−0.715	−7.535	0.000

[a] Dependent variable: PAF

The above table shows that treatment modality is weakly significant, and psychological and social scores are not. Furthermore, days of observation is very significant. However, it is not entirely appropriate to include this variable if your outcome is the numbers of events per person per time unit. Therefore, we will perform a linear regression, and adjust the outcome variable for the differences in days of observation using weighted least square regression.

Model		Coefficients[a,b]			t	Sig.
		Unstandardized coefficients		Standardized coefficients		
		B	Std. error	Beta		
1	(Constant)	10.033	2.862		3.506	0.001
	treat	−3.502	1.867	−0.269	−1.876	0.067
	psych	0.033	0.069	0.093	0.472	0.639
	soc	−0.093	0.078	−0.237	−1.194	0.238

[a] Dependent variable: PAF
[b] Weighted least squares regression—weighted by days

Command:
Analyze....Regression....Linear....Dependent: episodes of paroxysmal atrial fibrillation....Independent: treatment modality, psychological score, social score ....WLS Weight: days of observation.... OK.

The above table shows the results. A largely similar pattern is observed, but treatment modality is no more statistically significant. We will use the generalized linear modeling module to perform a Poisson regression which is more appropriate for rate data. The model applied will also be stored and reapplied for making predictions about event rates in individual future patients.

Command:
Click Transform....click Random Number Generators....click Set Starting Point.... click Fixed Value (2000000)....click OK....click Generalized Linear Models ....click again Generalized Linear Models....mark: Custom....Distribution: Poisson.....Link function: Log....Response: Dependent variable: numbers of episodes of PAF....Scale Weight Variable: days of observation....Predictors: Main Effect: treatment modality....Covariates: psychological score, social score.... Model: main effects: treatment modality, psychological score, social score.... Estimation: mark Model-based Estimation ....click Save....mark Predicted value of mean of response....click Export....mark Export model in XML....click Browse.... in File name enter "exportrate"....in Look in: enter the appropriate map in your computer for storage....click Save....click OK.

Parameter	B	Std. error	Parameter estimates					
			95 % Wald confidential interval		Hypothesis test			
			Lower	Upper	Wald Chi-square	df	Sig.	
(Intercept)	1.868	0.0206	1.828	1.909	8,256.274	1	0.000	
[treat = 0]	0.667	0.0153	0.637	0.697	1,897.429	1	0.000	
[treat = 1]	0^a							
psych	0.006	0.0006	0.005	0.008	120.966	1	0.000	
soc	−0.019	0.0006	−0.020	−0.017	830.264	1	0.000	
(Scale)	1^b							

Dependent variable: PAF
Model: (Intercept), treat, psych, soc
[a] Set to zero because this parameter is redundant
[b] Fixed at the displayed value

The outcome sheets give the results. All of a sudden, all of the predictors including treatment modality, psychological and social score are very significant predictors of the PAF rate. When minimizing the output sheets the data file returns and now shows a novel variable entitled "PredictedValues" with the mean rates of PAF episodes per patient (per day). The saved XML file will now be used to compute the predicted PAF rate in 5 novel patients with the following characteristics. For convenience the XML file is given in extras.springer.com.

Var 1	Var 2	Var 3	Var 4	Var 5
1.00	56.99	42.45	73.00	4.00
1.00	30.09	46.82	34.00	4.00
0.00	32.28	32.00	76.00	2.00
0.00	29.06	40.00	36.00	3.00
0.00	6.75	27.25	73.00	3.00

Var 1 = treatment modality
Var 2 = psychological score
Var 3 = social score
Var 4 = days of observation
Var 5 = number of episodes of paroxysmal atrial fibrillation (PAF) per day

Enter the above data in a new SPSS data file.

Command:
Utilities....click Scoring Wizard....click Browse....click Select....Folder: enter
the exportrate.xml file....click Select....in Scoring Wizard click Next....click Use
value substitution....click Next....click Finish.

The above data file now gives individually predicted rates of PAF as computed
by the linear model with the help of the XML file. Enter the above data in a new
SPSS data file.

Var 1	Var 2	Var 3	Var 4	Var 5	Var 6
1.00	56.99	42.45	73.00	4.00	4.23
1.00	30.09	46.82	34.00	4.00	3.27
0.00	32.28	32.00	76.00	2.00	8.54
0.00	29.06	40.00	36.00	3.00	7.20
0.00	6.75	27.25	73.00	3.00	7.92

Var 1 = treatment modality
Var 2 = psychological score
Var 3 = social score
Var 4 = days of observation
Var 5 = number of episodes of paroxysmal atrial fibrillation (PAF) per day
Var 6 = individually predicted mean rates of PAF (per day)

Conclusion

The module generalized linear models can be readily trained to predict event rate
of PAF episodes both in groups, and, with the help of an XML file, in individual
patients.

Note

More background, theoretical and mathematical information of generalized linear modeling is available in SPSS for Starters, Chap. 10, entitled "Poisson regression", pp. 43–48, Springer Heidelberg, Germany 2012.

Chapter 7
Factor Analysis and Partial Least Squares for Complex-Data Reduction (250 Patients)

General Purpose

A few unmeasured factors, otherwise called latent factors, are identified to explain a much larger number of measured factors, e.g., highly expressed chromosome-clustered genes. Unlike factor analysis, partial least squares (PLS) identifies not only exposure (x-value) but also outcome (y-value) variables.

Specific Scientific Question

Twelve highly expressed genes are used to predict drug efficacy. Is factor analysis/PLS better than traditional analysis for regression data with multiple exposure and outcome variables.

G1	G2	G3	G4	G16	G17	G18	G19	G24	G25	G26	G27	O1	O2	O3	O4
8	8	9	5	7	10	5	6	9	9	6	6	6	7	6	7
9	9	10	9	8	8	7	8	8	9	8	8	8	7	8	7
9	8	8	8	8	9	7	8	9	8	9	9	9	8	8	8
8	9	8	9	6	7	6	4	6	6	5	5	7	7	7	6
10	10	8	10	9	10	10	8	8	9	9	9	8	8	8	7
7	8	8	8	8	7	6	5	7	8	8	7	7	6	6	7
5	5	5	5	5	6	4	5	5	6	6	5	6	5	6	4
9	9	9	9	8	8	8	8	9	8	3	8	8	8	8	8
9	8	9	8	9	8	7	7	7	7	5	8	8	7	6	6
10	10	10	10	10	10	10	10	10	8	8	10	10	10	9	10
2	2	8	5	7	8	8	8	9	3	9	8	7	7	7	6

(continued)

T. J. Cleophas and A. H. Zwinderman, *Machine Learning in Medicine - Cookbook*, SpringerBriefs in Statistics, DOI: 10.1007/978-3-319-04181-0_7, © The Author(s) 2014

(continued)

G1	G2	G3	G4	G16	G17	G18	G19	G24	G25	G26	G27	O1	O2	O3	O4
7	8	8	7	8	6	6	7	8	8	8	7	8	7	8	8
8	9	9	8	10	8	8	7	8	8	9	9	7	7	8	8

Var G1–27 = highly expressed genes estimated from their arrays' normalized ratios
Var O1–4 = drug efficacy scores (the variables 20–23 from the initial data file)
The data from the first 13 patients are shown only (see extras.springer.com for the entire data file
entitled "optscalingfactorplscanonical")

Factor Analysis

First the reliability of the model was assessed by assessing the test–retest reliability
of the original predictor variables using the correlation coefficients after deletion
of one variable: all of the data files should produce at least by 80 % the same result
as that of the non-deleted data file (alphas > 80 %). SPSS 19.0 is used. Start by
opening the data file.

Command:
Analyze....Scale....Reliability Analysis....transfer original variables to Variables
box....click Statistics....mark Scale if item deleted....mark Correlations
....Continue....OK.

Item-total statistics					
	Scale mean if item deleted	Scale variance if item deleted	Corrected item-total correlation	Squared multiple correlation	Cronbach's alpha if item deleted
Geneone	80.8680	276.195	0.540	0.485	0.902
Genetwo	80.8680	263.882	0.700	0.695	0.895
Genethree	80.7600	264.569	0.720	0.679	0.895
Genefour	80.7960	282.002	0.495	0.404	0.904
Genesixteen	81.6200	258.004	0.679	0.611	0.896
Geneseventeen	80.9800	266.196	0.680	0.585	0.896
Geneeighteen	81.5560	263.260	0.606	0.487	0.899
Genenineteen	82.2040	255.079	0.696	0.546	0.895
Genetwentyfour	81.5280	243.126	0.735	0.632	0.893
Genetwentyfive	81.2680	269.305	0.538	0.359	0.902
Genetwentysix	81.8720	242.859	0.719	0.629	0.894
Genetwentyseven	81.0720	264.501	0.540	0.419	0.903

None of the original variables after deletion reduce the test–retest reliability. The data are reliable. We will now perform the principal components analysis with three components, otherwise called latent variables.

Command:
Analyze....Dimension Reduction....Factor....enter variables into Variables box....click Extraction....Method: click Principle Components....mark Correlation Matrix, Unrotated factor solution....Fixed number of factors: enter 3....Maximal Iterations plot Convergence: enter 25....Continue....click Rotation....Method: click Varimax....mark Rotated solution....mark Loading Plots....Maximal Iterations: enter 25....Continue....click Scores.... mark Display factor score coefficient matrix ....OK.

Rotated component matrix[a]

	Component		
	1	2	3
Geneone	0.211	0.810	0.143
Genetwo	0.548	0.683	0.072
Genethree	0.624	0.614	0.064
Genefour	0.033	0.757	0.367
Genesixteen	0.857	0.161	0.090
Geneseventeen	0.650	0.216	0.338
Geneeighteen	0.526	0.297	0.318
Genenineteen	0.750	0.266	0.170
Genetwentyfour	0.657	0.100	0.539
Genetwentyfive	0.219	0.231	0.696
Genetwentysix	0.687	0.077	0.489
Genetwentyseven	0.188	0.159	0.825

Extraction method: principal component analysis
Rotation method: Varimax with Kaiser normalization
[a] Rotation converged in 8 iterations

The best fit coefficients of the original variables constituting 3 new factors (unmeasured, otherwise called latent, factors) are given. The latent factor 1 has a very strong correlation with the genes 16–19, the latent factor 2 with the genes 1–4, and the latent factor 3 with the genes 24–27.

When returning to the data file, we now observe, that, for each patient, the software program has produced the individual values of these novel predictors.

In order to fit these novel predictors with the outcome variables, the drug efficacy scores (variables O1–4), multivariate analysis of variance (MANOVA) should be appropriate. However, the large number of columns in the design matrix caused integer overflow, and the command was not executed. Instead we will perform a univariate multiple linear regression with the add-up scores of the outcome variables (using the Transform and Compute Variable command) as novel outcome variable.

Command:
Transform....Compute Variable....transfer outcomeone to Numeric Expression box....click+....outcometwo idem....click+....outcomethree idem....click+.... outcomefour idem....Target Variable: enter "summaryoutcome"....click OK.

In the data file the summaryoutcome values are displayed as a novel variable (variable 28).

Command:
Analyze....Regression....Dependent: enter summaryoutcome....Independent: enter Fac 1, Fac 2, and Fac 3....click OK.

Coefficients[a]

Model	Unstandardized coefficients		Standardized coefficients	t	Sig.
	B	Std. error	Bela		
1 (Constant)	27.332	0.231		118.379	0.000
REGR factor score 1 for analysis 1	5.289	0.231	0.775	22.863	0.000
REGR factor score 2 for analysis 1	1.749	0.231	0.256	7.562	0.000
REGR factor score 3 for analysis 1	1.529	0.231	0.224	6.611	0.000

[a] Dependent variable: summaryoutcome

All of the 3 latent predictors were, obviously, very significant predictors of the summary outcome variable.

Partial Least Squares Analysis

Because Partial least squares analysis (PLS) is not available in the basic and regression modules of SPSS, the software program R Partial Least Squares, a free statistics and forecasting software available on the internet as a free online software calculator was used (www.wessa.net/rwasp). The data file is imported directly from the SPSS file entitled "optscalingfactorplscanonical" (cut/past commands).

Command:
List the selected clusters of variables: latent variable 2 (here G16–19), latent variable 1 (here G24–27), latent variable 4 (here G1–4), and latent outcome variable 3 (here O1–4).

A square boolean matrix is constructed with "0 or 1" values if fitted correlation coefficients to be included in the model were "no or yes" according to the underneath table.

Latent variable		1	2	3	4
Latent variable	1	0	0	0	0
	2	0	0	0	0
	3	1	1	0	0
	4	0	0	1	0

Click "compute". After 15 s of computing the program produces the results. First, the data were validated using the goodness of fit (GoF) criteria. GoF $= \sqrt{}$ [mean of r-square values of comparisons in model * r-square overall model], where * is the sign of multiplication. A GoF value varies from 0 to 1 and values larger than 0.8 indicate that the data are adequately reliable for modeling.

GoF value	
Overall	0.9459
Outer model (including manifest variables)	0.9986
Inner model (including latent variables)	0.9466

The data are, thus, adequately reliable. The calculated best fit r-values (correlation coefficients) are estimated from the model, and their standard errors would be available from second derivatives. However, the problem with the second derivatives is that they require very large data files in order to be accurate. Instead, distribution free standard errors are calculated using bootstrap resampling.

Latent variables	Original r-value	Bootstrap r-value	Standard error	t-value
1 versus 3	0.57654	0.57729	0.08466	6.8189
2 versus 3	0.67322	0.67490	0.04152	16.2548
4 versus 3	0.18322	0.18896	0.05373	3.5168

All of the three correlation coefficients (r-values) are very significant predictors of the latent outcome variable.

Traditional Linear Regression

When using the summary scores of the main components of the 3 latent variables instead of the above modeled latent variables (using the above Transform and Compute Variable commands), the effects remained statistically significant, however, at lower levels of significance.

Command:
Analyze....Regression....Linear....Dependent: enter summaryoutcome.... Independent: enter the three summary factors 1–3....click OK.

Coefficients[a]

Model	Unstandardized coefficients		Standardized coefficients	t	Sig.
	B	Std. error	Beta		
1 (Constant)	1.177	1.407		0.837	0.404
Summaryfacl	0.136	0.059	0.113	2.316	0.021
Summaryfac2	0.620	0.054	0.618	11.413	0.000
Summaryfac3	0.150	0.044	0.170	3.389	0.001

[a] Dependent variable: summaryoutcome

The partial least squares method produces smaller t-values than did factor analysis (t = 3.5–16.3 versus 6.6–22.9), but it is less biased, because it is a multivariate analysis adjusting relationships between the outcome variables. Both methods provided better t-values than did the above traditional regression analysis of summary variables (t = 2.3–11.4).

Conclusion

Factor analysis and PLS can handle many more variables than the standard methods, and account the relative importance of the separate variables, their interactions and differences in units. Partial least squares method is parsimonious to principal components analysis because it can separately include outcome variables in the model.

Note

More background, theoretical and mathematical information of the three methods is given in Machine Learning in Medicine Part one, Chaps. 14 and 16, Factor analysis pp. 167–181, and Partial least squares, pp. 197–212, Springer Heidelberg Germany 2013.

Chapter 8
Optimal Scaling of High-Sensitivity Analysis of Health Predictors (250 Patients)

General Purpose

In linear models of health predictors (x-values) and health outcomes (y-values), better power of testing can sometimes be obtained, if continuous predictor variables are converted into the best fit discretized ones.

Specific Scientific Question

Highly expressed genes were used to predict drug efficacy. The example from Chap. 7 was used once more. The gene expression levels were scored on a scale of 0–10, but some scores were rarely observed. Can the strength of prediction be improved by optimal scaling.

G1	G2	G3	G4	G16	G17	G18	G19	G24	G25	G26	G27	O1	O2	O3	O4
8	8	9	5	7	10	5	6	9	9	6	6	6	7	6	7
9	9	10	9	8	8	7	8	8	9	8	8	8	7	8	7
9	8	8	8	8	9	7	8	9	8	9	9	9	8	8	8
8	9	8	9	6	7	6	4	6	6	5	5	7	7	7	6
10	10	8	10	9	10	10	8	8	9	9	9	8	8	8	7
7	8	8	8	8	7	6	5	7	8	8	7	7	6	6	7
5	5	5	5	5	6	4	5	5	6	6	5	6	5	6	4
9	9	9	9	8	8	8	8	9	8	3	8	8	8	8	8
9	8	9	8	9	8	7	7	7	7	5	8	8	7	6	6
10	10	10	10	10	10	10	10	10	8	8	10	10	10	9	10

(continued)

T. J. Cleophas and A. H. Zwinderman, *Machine Learning in Medicine - Cookbook*, SpringerBriefs in Statistics, DOI: 10.1007/978-3-319-04181-0_8, © The Author(s) 2014

(continued)

G1	G2	G3	G4	G16	G17	G18	G19	G24	G25	G26	G27	O1	O2	O3	O4
2	2	8	5	7	8	8	8	9	3	9	8	7	7	7	6
7	8	8	7	8	6	6	7	8	8	8	7	8	7	8	8
8	9	9	8	10	8	8	7	8	8	9	9	7	7	8	8

Var G1–27 = highly expressed genes estimated from their arrays' normalized ratios
Var O1–4 = drug efficacy scores which are the variables 20–23 from the initial data file (sum of the scores is used as outcome)
Only the data from the first 13 patients are shown. The entire data file entitled "optscalingfactorplscanonical" can be downloaded from extra.springer.com

Traditional Multiple Linear Regression

SPSS 19.0 is used for data analysis. Open the data file and command.

Command:
Transform....Compute Variable....transfer outcomeone to Numeric Expression box....click+....outcometwo idem....click+....outcomethree idem....click+....outcomefour idem....Target Variable: enter "summaryoutcome"....click OK.

In the data file the summaryoutcome values are displayed as a novel variable (variable 28).

Command:
Analyze....Regression....Linear....Independent: enter the 12 highly expressed genes....Dependent: enter the summary scores of the 4 outcome variables....click OK.

Coefficients[a]					
Model	Unstandardized coefficients		Standardized coefficients	t	Sig.
	B	Std. error	Beta		
1 (Constant)	3.293	1.475		2.232	0.027
geneone	−0.122	0.189	−0.030	−0.646	0.519
genetwo	0.287	0.225	0.3078	1.276	0.203
genethree	0.370	0.228	0.097	1.625	0.105
genefour	0.063	0.196	0.014	0.321	0.748
genesixteen	0.764	0.172	0.241	4.450	0.000
geneseventeen	0.835	0.198	0.221	4.220	0.000
geneeighteen	0.088	0.151	0.027	0.580	0.563
genenineteen	0.576	0.154	0.188	3.751	0.000
genetwentyfour	0.403	0.146	0.154	2.760	0.006
genetwentyfive	0.028	0.141	0.008	0.198	0.843

(continued)

(continued)

Coefficients[a]

Model	Unstandardized coefficients		Standardized coefficients	t	Sig.
	B	Std. error	Beta		
genetwentysix	0.320	0.142	0.125	2.250	0.025
genetwentyseven	−0.275	0.133	−0.092	−2.067	0.040

[a] Dependent variable: summaryoutcome

The number of statistically significant p-values (indicated here with Sig.), (<0.10) was 6 out of 12. In order to improve this result the Optimal Scaling program of SPSS is used. Continuous predictor variables are converted into best fit discretized ones.

Optimal Scaling Without Regularization

Command:
Analyze....Regression....Optimal Scaling....Dependent Variable: Var 28 (Define Scale: mark spline ordinal 2.2)....Independent Variables: Var 1, 2, 3, 4, 16, 17, 18, 19, 24, 25, 26, 27 (all of them Define Scale: mark spline ordinal 2.2)....Discretize: Method Grouping)....OK.

Coefficients[a]

	Standardized coefficients		df	F	Sig.
	Beta	Bootstrap (1,000) estimate of std. error			
geneone	−0.109	0.110	2	0.988	0.374
genetwo	0.193	0.107	3	3.250	0.023
genethree	−0.092	0.119	2	0.591	0.555
genefour	0.113	0.074	3	2.318	0.077
genesixteen	0.263	0.087	4	9.065	0.000
geneseventeen	0.301	0.114	2	6.935	0.001
geneeighteen	0.113	0.136	1	0.687	0.408
genenineteen	0.145	0.067	1	4.727	0.031
genetwentyfour	0.220	0.097	2	5.166	0.007
genetwentyfive	−0.039	0.094	1	0.170	0.681
genetwentysix	0.058	0.107	2	0.293	0.746
genetwentyseven	−0.127	0.104	2	1.490	0.228

[a] Dependent variable: summaryoutcome

There is no intercept anymore and the t-tests have been replaced with F-tests. The optimally scaled model without regularization shows similarly sized effects.

The number of *p*-values <0.10 is 6 out of 12. In order to fully benefit from optimal scaling a regularization procedure for the purpose of correcting overdispersion (more spread in the data than compatible with Gaussian data) is desirable. Ridge regression minimizes the b-values such that $b_{ridge} = b/(1 + shrinking factor)$. With shrinking factor = 0, $b_{ridge} = b$, with ∞, $b_{ridge} = 0$.

Optimal Scaling with Ridge Regression

Command:
Analyze....Regression....Optimal Scaling....Dependent Variable: Var 28 (Define Scale: mark spline ordinal 2.2)....Independent Variables: Var 1, 2, 3, 4, 16, 17, 18, 19, 24, 25, 26, 27 (all of them Define Scale: mark spline ordinal 2.2)....Discretize: Method Grouping, Number categories 7)....click Regularization....mark Ridge.... OK.

Coefficients[a]

| | Standardized coefficients | | df | F | Sig. |
	Beta	Bootstrap (1,000) estimate of std. error			
geneone	0.032	0.033	2	0.946	0.390
genetwo	0.068	0.021	3	10.842	0.000
genethree	0.051	0.030	1	2.963	0.087
genefour	0.064	0.020	3	10.098	0.000
genesixteen	0.139	0.024	4	34.114	0.000
geneseventeen	0.142	0.025	2	31.468	0.000
geneeighteen	0.108	0.040	2	7.236	0.001
genenineteen	0.109	0.020	2	30.181	0.000
genetwentyfour	0.109	0.021	2	27.855	0.000
genetwenlyfive	0.041	0.038	3	1.178	0.319
genetwentysix	0.098	0.023	2	17.515	0.000
genetwentyseven	−0.017	0.047	1	0.132	0.716

[a] Dependent variable: 20–23

The sensitivity of this model is better than the above two methods with 7 *p*-values <0.0001, and 9 *p*-values <0.10, while the traditional and unregularized Optimal Scaling only produced 6 and 6 *p*-values <0.10. Also the lasso regularization model is possible (Var = variable). It shrinks the small b values to 0.

Optimal Scaling with Lasso Regression

Command:
Analyze....Regression....Optimal Scaling....Dependent Variable: Var 28 (Define Scale: mark spline ordinal 2.2)....Independent Variables: Var 1, 2, 3, 4, 16, 17, 18,

19, 24, 25, 26, 27 (all of them Define Scale: mark spline ordinal 2.2)….Discretize: Method Grouping, Number categories 7)….click Regularization….mark Lasso…. OK.

Coefficients[a]

	Standardized coefficients		df	F	Sip.
	Beta	Bootstrap (1,000) estimate of std. error			
geneone	0.000	0.020	0	0.000	
genetwo	0.054	0.046	3	1.390	0.247
genethree	0.000	0.026	0	0.000	
genefour	0.011	0.036	3	0.099	0.960
genesixteen	0.182	0.084	4	4.684	0.001
geneseventeen	0.219	0.095	3	5.334	0.001
geneeighteen	0.086	0.079	2	1.159	0.316
genenineteen	0.105	0.063	2	2.803	0.063
genetwentyfour	0.124	0.078	2	2.532	0.082
genetwentyfive	0.000	0.023	0	0.000	
genetwentysix	0.048	0.060	2	0.647	0.525
genetwentyseven	0.000	0.022	0	0.000	

[a] Dependent variable: 20–23

The b-values of the genes 1, 3, 25 and 27 are now shrunk to zero, and eliminated from the analysis. Lasso is particularly suitable if you are looking for a limited number of predictors and improves prediction accuracy by leaving out weak predictors. Finally, the elastic net method is applied. Like lasso it shrinks the small b-values to 0, but it performs better with many predictor variables.

Optimal Scaling with Elastic Net Regression

Command:
Analyze….Regression….Optimal Scaling….Dependent Variable: Var 28 (Define Scale: mark spline ordinal 2.2)….Independent Variables: Var 1, 2, 3, 4, 16, 17, 18, 19, 24, 25, 26, 27 (all of them Define Scale: mark spline ordinal 2.2)….Discretize: Method Grouping, Number categories 7)….click Regularization….mark Elastic Net….OK.

Coefficients[a]

	Standardized coefficients		df	F	Sig.
	Beta	Bootstrap (1,000) estimate of std. error			
geneone	0.000	0.016	0	0.000	

(continued)

(continued)

Coefficients[a]

	Standardized coefficients		df	F	Sig.
	Beta	Bootstrap (1,000) estimate of std. error			
genetwo	0.029	0.039	3	0.553	0.647
genethree	0.000	0.032	3	0.000	1.000
genefour	0.000	0.015	0	0.000	
genesixteen	0.167	0.048	4	12.265	0.000
geneseventeen	0.174	0.051	3	11.429	0.000
geneeighteen	0.105	0.055	2	3.598	0.029
genenineteen	0.089	0.048	3	3.420	0.018
genetwentyfour	0.113	0.053	2	4.630	0.011
genetwenlyfive	0.000	0.012	0	0.000	
genetwentysix	0.062	0.046	2	1.786	0.170
genetwentyseven	0.000	0.018	0	0.000	

[a] Dependent variable: 20–23

The results are pretty much the same, as it is with lasso. Elastic net does not provide additional benefit in this example but works better than lasso if the number of predictors is larger than the number of observations.

Conclusion

Optimal scaling of linear regression data provides little benefit due to overdispersion. Regularized optimal scaling using ridge regression provides excellent results. Lasso optimal scaling is suitable if you are looking for a limited number of strong predictors. Elastic net optimal scaling works better than lasso if the number of predictors is large.

Note

More background, theoretical and mathematical information of optimal scaling with or without regularization is available in Machine Learning in Medicine Part One, Chaps. 3 and 4, entitled "Optimal scaling: discretization", and "Optimal scaling: regularization including ridge, lasso, and elastic net regression", pp. 25–37, and pp. 39–53, Springer Heidelberg Germany 2013.

Chapter 9
Discriminant Analysis for Making a Diagnosis from Multiple Outcomes (45 Patients)

General Purpose

To assess whether discriminant analysis can be used to make a diagnosis from multiple outcomes both in groups and in individual patients.

Specific Scientific Question

Laboratory screenings were performed in patients with different types of sepsis (urosepsis, bile duct sepsis, and airway sepsis). Can discriminant analysis of laboratory screenings improve reliability of diagnostic processes.

Var 1	Var 2	Var 3	Var 4	Var 5	Var 6	Var 7	Var 8	Var 9	Var 10	Var 11
8.00	5.00	28.00	4.00	2.50	79.00	108.00	19.00	18.00	16.00	2.00
11.00	10.00	29.00	7.00	2.10	94.00	89.00	18.00	15.00	15.00	2.00
7.00	8.00	30.00	7.00	2.20	79.00	96.00	20.00	16.00	14.00	2.00
4.00	6.00	16.00	6.00	2.60	80.00	120.00	17.00	17.00	19.00	2.00
1.00	6.00	15.00	6.00	2.20	84.00	108.00	21.00	18.00	20.00	2.00
23.00	5.00	14.00	6.00	2.10	78.00	120.00	18.00	17.00	21.00	3.00
12.00	10.00	17.00	5.00	3.20	85.00	100.00	17.00	20.00	18.00	3.00
31.00	8.00	27.00	5.00	0.20	68.00	113.00	19.00	15.00	18.00	3.00
22.00	7.00	26.00	5.00	1.20	74.00	98.00	16.00	16.00	17.00	3.00
30.00	6.00	25.00	4.00	2.40	69.00	90.00	20.00	18.00	16.00	3.00

(continued)

T. J. Cleophas and A. H. Zwinderman, *Machine Learning in Medicine - Cookbook*, SpringerBriefs in Statistics, DOI: 10.1007/978-3-319-04181-0_9, © The Author(s) 2014

(continued)

Var 1	Var 2	Var 3	Var 4	Var 5	Var 6	Var 7	Var 8	Var 9	Var 10	Var 11
2.00	12.00	21.00	4.00	2.80	75.00	112.00	11.00	14.00	19.00	1.00
10.00	21.00	20.00	4.00	2.90	70.00	100.00	12.00	15.00	20.00	1.00

Var 1 = gammagt
Var 2 = asat
Var 3 = alat
Var 4 = bilirubine
Var 5 = ureum
Var 6 = creatinine
Var 7 = creatinine clearance
Var 8 = erythrocyte sedimentation rate
Var 9 = c-reactive protein
Var 10 = leucocyte count
Var 11 = type of sepsis (1–3 as described above)
The first 12 patients are shown only, the entire data file is entitled "discriminant analysis" and is in extras.springer.com

The Computer Teaches Itself to Make Predictions

SPSS 19.0 is used for training and outcome prediction. It uses XML (eXtended Markup Language) file to store data. Start by opening the data file.

Command
Click Transform....click Random Number generator Generators....click Set Starting Point.... click Fixed Value (2000000)....click OK....click Analyze....Classify.... Discriminant Analysis....Grouping Variable: enter diagnosis group....Define Range: Minimum enter 1...Maximum enter 3....click Continue....Independents: enter all of the 10 laboratory variables....click Statistics....mark Unstandardized ....mark Separate-groups covariance....click Continue....click Classify....mark All groups equal....mark Summary table....-mark Within-groups....mark Combined groups....click Continue....click Save....mark Predicted group memberships....in Export model information to XML file enter: export discriminant....click Browse and save the XML file in your computer....click Continue....click OK.

The scientific question "is the diagnosis group a significant predictor of the outcome estimated with 10 lab values" is hard to assess with traditional multivariate methods due to interaction between the outcome variables. It is, therefore, assessed with the question "is the clinical outcome a significant predictor of the odds of having had a particular prior diagnosis". This reasoning may seem incorrect, using an outcome for making predictions, but, mathematically, it is no problem. It is just a matter of linear cause-effect relationships, but just the other way around, and it works very conveniently with "messy" outcome variables like in the example given. However, first, the numbers of outcome variables have to be reduced. SPSS accomplishes this by orthogonal modeling of the outcome

variables, which produces novel composite outcome variables. They are the
y-values of linear equations. The x-values of these linear equations are the original
outcome variables, and their regression coefficients are given in the underneath
table.

Structure Matrix		
	Function	
	1	2
As at	0.574[a]	0.184
Gammagt	0.460[a]	0.203
C-reactive protein	−0.034	0.761[a]
Leucos	0.193	0.537[a]
Ureum	0.461	0.533[a]
Creatinine	0.0462	0.520[a]
Alat	0.411	0.487[a]
Bili	0.356	0.487[a]
Esr	0.360	0.487[a]
Creatinine clearance	−0.083	−0.374[a]

Pooled within-groups correlations between discriminating variables and standardized canonical
discriminant functions
Variables ordered by absolute size of correlation within function
[a] Largest absolute correlation between each variable and any discriminant function

Wilks' Lambda				
Test of Function(s)	Wilks' Lambda	Chi square	df	Sig.
1 through 2	0.420	32.500	20	0.038
2	0.859	5.681	9	0.771

The two novel outcome variables significantly predict the odds of having had a
prior diagnosis with $p = 0.038$ as shown above. When minimizing the output
sheets we will return to the data file and observe that the novel outcome variables
have been added (the variables entitled Dis1_1 and Dis1_2), as well as the predicted diagnosis group predicted from the discriminant model (the variable entitled
Dis_1). For convenience the XML file entitled "export discriminant" is stored in
extras.springer.com.

The saved XML file can now be used to predict the odds of having been in a
particular diagnosis group in five novel patients whose lab values are known but
whose diagnoses are not yet obvious.

Var 1	Var 2	Var 3	Var 4	Var 5	Var 6	Var 7	Var 8	Var 9	Var 10
1,049.00	466.00	301.00	268.00	59.80	213.00	−2.00	109.00	121.00	42.00
383.00	230.00	154.00	120.00	31.80	261.00	13.00	80.00	58.00	30.00
9.00	9.00	31.00	204.00	34.80	222.00	10.00	60.00	57.00	34.00
438.00	391.00	479.00	127.00	31.80	372.00	9.00	69.00	56.00	33.00
481.00	348.00	478.00	139.00	21.80	329.00	15.00	49.00	47.00	32.00

Var 1 = gammagt
Var 2 = asat
Var 3 = alat
Var 4 = bilirubine
Var 5 = ureum
Var 6 = creatinine
Var 7 = creatinine clearance
Var 8 = erythrocyte sedimentation rate
Var 9 = c-reactive protein
Var 10 = leucocyte count

Enter the above data in a new SPSS data file.

Command:
Utilities....click Scoring Wizard....click Browse....click Select....Folder: enter the exportdiscriminant.xml file....click Select....in Scoring Wizard click Next....click Use value substitution....click Next....click Finish.

The above data file now gives predicted odds of having been in a particular diagnosis group computed by the discriminant analysis module with the help of the xml file.

Var 1	Var 2	Var 3	Var 4	Var 5	Var 6	Var 7	Var 8	Var 9	Var 10	Var 11
1,049.00	466.00	301.00	268.00	59.80	213.00	−2.00	109.00	121.00	42.00	2.00
383.00	230.00	154.00	120.00	31.80	261.00	13.00	80.00	58.00	30.00	2.00
9.00	9.00	31.00	204.00	34.80	222.00	10.00	60.00	57.00	34.00	1.00
438.00	391.00	479.00	127.00	31.80	372.00	9.00	69.00	56.00	33.00	1.00
481.00	348.00	478.00	139.00	21.80	329.00	15.00	49.00	47.00	32.00	2.00

Var 1 = gammagt
Var 2 = asat
Var 3 = alat
Var 4 = bilirubine
Var 5 = ureum
Var 6 = creatinine
Var 7 = creatinine clearance
Var 8 = erythrocyte sedimentation rate
Var 9 = c-reactive protein
Var 10 = leucocyte count
Var 11 = predicted odds of having been in a particular diagnosis group

Conclusion

The discriminant analysis module can be readily trained to provide from the laboratory values of individual patients the best fit odds of having been in a particular diagnosis group. In this way discriminant analysis can support the hard work of physicians trying to make a diagnosis.

Note

More background, theoretical and mathematical information of discriminant analysis is available in Machine Learning Part One, Chap. 17, entitled "Discriminant analysis for supervised data ", pp. 215–224, Springer Heidelberg Germany 2013.

Chapter 10
Weighted Least Squares for Adjusting Efficacy Data with Inconsistent Spread (78 Patients)

General Purpose

Linear regression assumes that the spread of the outcome-values is homoscedastic: it is the same for each predictor value. This assumption is, however, not warranted in many real life situations. This chapter is to assess the advantages of *weighted* least squares (WLS) instead of *ordinary* least squares (OLS) linear regression analysis.

Specific Scientific Question

The effect of prednisone on peak expiratory flow was assumed to be more variable with increasing dosages. Can it, therefore, be measured with more precision if linear regression is replaced with weighted least squares procedure.

Var 1	Var 2	Var 3	Var 4
1	29	1.40	174
2	15	2.00	113
3	38	0.00	281
4	26	1.00	127
5	47	1.00	267
6	28	0.20	172
7	20	2.00	118
8	47	0.40	383
9	39	0.40	97
10	43	1.60	304
11	16	0.40	85
12	35	1.80	182
13	47	2.00	140

(continued)

T. J. Cleophas and A. H. Zwinderman, *Machine Learning in Medicine - Cookbook*, SpringerBriefs in Statistics, DOI: 10.1007/978-3-319-04181-0_10, © The Author(s) 2014

(continued)

Var 1	Var 2	Var 3	Var 4
14	35	2.00	64
15	38	0.20	153
16	40	0.40	216

Var 1 = patient no
Var 2 = prednisone (mg/24 h)
Var 3 = peak flow (ml/min)
Var 4 = beta agonist (mg/24 h)

Only the first 16 patients are given, the entire data file is entitled "weighted-leastsquares" and is in extras.springer.com. SPSS 19.0 is used for data analysis. We will first make a graph of prednisone dosages and peak expiratory flows. Start with opening the data file.

Weighted Least Squares

Command:
click Graphs....Legacy Dialogs....Scatter/Dot....click Simple Scatter....click Define....Y Axis enter peakflow....X Axis enter prednisone....click OK.

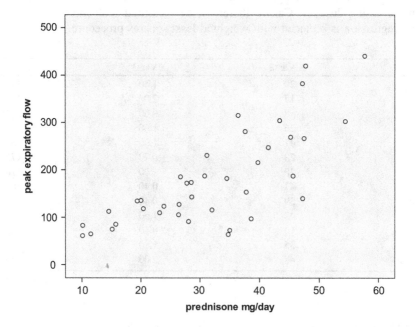

The output sheet shows that the spread of the y-values is small with low dosages and gradually increases. We will, therefore, perform both a traditional and a weighted least squares analysis of these data.

Command:
Analyze....Regression....Linear....Dependent: enter peakflow....
Independent: enter prednisone, betaagonist....OK.

Model summary[b]				
Model	R	R square	Adjusted R square	Std. error of the estimate
1	0.763[a]	0.582	0.571	65.304

[a] Predictors: (Constant), beta agonist mg/24 h, prednisone mg/day
[b] Dependent variable: peak expiratory flow

Coefficients[a]					
Model	Unstandardized coefficients		Standardized coefficients	t	Sig.
	B	Std. error	Beta		
1 (Constant)	−22.534	22.235		−1.013	0.314
Prednisone mg/day	6.174	0.604	0.763	10.217	0.000
Beta agonist mg/24 h	6.744	11.299	0.045	0.597	0.552

[a] Dependent variable: peak expiratory flow

In the output sheets an R value of 0.763 is observed, and the linear effects of prednisone dosages are a statistically significant predictor of the peak expiratory flow, but, surprisingly, the beta agonists dosages are not.

We will, subsequently, perform a WLS analysis.

Command:
Analyze....Regression....Weight Estimation.... select: Dependent: enter peakflow .... Independent(s): enter prednisone, betaagonist....select prednisone also as Weight variable....Power range: enter 0 through 5 by 0.5....click Options....select Save best weights as new variable....click Continue....click OK.

In the output sheets it is observed that the software has calculated likelihoods for different powers, and the best likelihood value is chosen for further analysis. When returning to the data file again a novel variable is added, the WGT_1 variable (the weights for the WLS analysis). The next step is to perform again a linear regression, but now with the weight variable included.

Command:
Analyze....Regression....Linear.... select: Dependent: enter peakflow.... Independent(s) : enter prednisone, betaagonist....select the weights for the wls analysis (the WGT_1) variable as WLS Weight....click Save....select Unstandardized in Predicted Values....deselect Standardized in Residuals....click Continue....click OK.

Model Summary[b,c]

Model	R	R square	Adjusted R square	Std. error of the estimate
1	0.846[a]	0.716	0.709	0.125

[a] Predictors: (Constant), beta agonist mg/24 h, prednisone mg/day
[b] Dependent variable: peak expiratory flow
[c] Weighted least squares regression: Weighted by weight for peakflow from WLS, MOD_6 PREDNISONE**-3.500

Coefficients[a,b]

Model	Unstandardized coefficients		Standardized coefficients	t	Sig.
	B	Std. error	Beta		
1 (Constant)	5.029	7.544		0.667	0.507
Prednisone mg/day	5.064	0.369	0.880	13.740	0.000
Beta agonist mg/24 h	10.838	3.414	0.203	3.174	0.002

[a] Dependent variable: peak expiratory flow
[b] Weighted least squares regression: Weighted by weight for peakflow from WLS, MOD_6 PREDNISONE**-3.500

The output table now shows an R value of 0.846. It has risen from 0.763, and provides thus more statistical power. The above lower table shows the effects of the two medicine dosages on the peak expiratory flows. The t-values of the medicine predictors have increased from approximately 10 and 0.5 to 14 and 3.2. The p-values correspondingly fell from 0.000 and 0.552 to respectively 0.000 and 0.002. Larger prednisone dosages and larger beta agonist dosages significantly and independently increased peak expiratory flows. After adjustment for heteroscedasticity, the beta agonist became a significant independent determinant of peak flow.

Conclusion

The current paper shows that, even with a sample of only 78 patients, WLS is able to demonstrate statistically significant linear effects that had been, previously, obscured by heteroscedasticity of the y-value.

Note

More background, theoretical and mathematical information of weighted least squares modeling is given in Machine Learning in Medicine Part Three, Chap. 10, Weighted least squares, pp 107–116, Springer Heidelberg Germany 2013.

Chapter 11
Partial Correlations for Removing Interaction Effects from Efficacy Data (64 Patients)

General Purpose

The outcome of cardiovascular research is generally affected by many more factors than a single one, and multiple regression assumes that these factors act independently of one another, but why should they not affect one another. This chapter is to assess whether partial correlation can be used to remove interaction effects from linear data.

Specific Scientific Question

Both calorie intake and exercise are significant independent predictors of weight loss. However, exercise makes you hungry and patients on weight training are inclined to reduce (or increase) their calorie intake. Can partial correlations methods adjust the interaction between the two predictors.

Var 1	Var 2	Var 3	Var 4	Var 5
1.00	0.00	1,000.00	0.00	45.00
29.00	0.00	1,000.00	0.00	53.00
2.00	0.00	3,000.00	0.00	64.00
1.00	0.00	3,000.00	0.00	64.00
28.00	6.00	3,000.00	18,000.00	34.00
27.00	6.00	3,000.00	18,000.00	25.00
30.00	6.00	3,000.00	18,000.00	34.00
27.00	6.00	1,000.00	6,000.00	45.00
29.00	0.00	2,000.00	0.00	52.00
31.00	3.00	2,000.00	6,000.00	59.00
30.00	3.00	1,000.00	3,000.00	58.00
29.00	3.00	1,000.00	3,000.00	47.00

(continued)

T. J. Cleophas and A. H. Zwinderman, *Machine Learning in Medicine - Cookbook*, SpringerBriefs in Statistics, DOI: 10.1007/978-3-319-04181-0_11, © The Author(s) 2014

(continued)

Var 1	Var 2	Var 3	Var 4	Var 5
27.00	0.00	1,000.00	0.00	45.00
28.00	0.00	1,000.00	0.00	66.00
27.00	0.00	1,000.00	0.00	67.00

Var 1 = weight loss (kg)
Var 2 = exercise (times per week)
Var 3 = calorie intake (cal)
Var 4 = interaction
Var 5 = age (years)

Only the first fifteen patients are given, the entire file is entitled "partialcorrelations" and is in extras.springer.com.

Partial Correlations

We will first perform a linear regression of these data. SPSS 19.0 is used for the purpose. Start by opening the data file.

Command:
Analyze....Regression....Linear....Dependent variable: enter weightloss.... Independent variables: enter exercise and calorieintake....click OK.

Coefficients[a]

Model	Unstandardized coefficients		Standardized coefficients	t	Sig.
	B	Std. error	Beta		
1 (Constant)	29.089	2.241		12.978	0.000
Exercise	2.548	0.439	0.617	5.802	0.000
Calorieintake	−0.006	0.001	−0.544	−5.116	0.000

[a] Dependent variable: weightloss

The output sheets show that both calorie intake and exercise are significant independent predictors of weight loss. However, interaction between exercise and calorie intake is not accounted. In order to check, an interaction variable (x_3 = calorie intake * exercise, with * symbol of multiplication) is added to the model.

Command:
Transform data....Compute Variable....in Target Variable enter the term "interaction"....to Numeric Expression: transfer from Type & Label "exercise" ....click * ....transfer from Type & Label calorieintake....click OK.

The interaction variable is added by SPSS to the data file and is entitled "interaction". After the addition of the interaction variable to the regression model as third independent variable, the analysis is repeated.

Coefficients[a]

Model	Unstandardized coefficients		Standardized coefficients	t	Sig.
	B	Std. error	Beta		
1 (Constant)	34.279	2.651		12.930	0.000
Interaction	0.001	0.000	0.868	3.183	0.002
Exercise	−0.238	0.966	−0.058	−0.246	0.807
Calorieintake	−0.009	0.002	−0.813	−6.240	0.000

[a] Dependent variable: weightloss

The output sheet now shows that exercise is no longer significant and interaction on the outcome is significant at $p = 0.002$. There is, obviously, interaction in the study, and the overall analysis of the data is, thus, no longer relevant. The best method to find the true effect of exercise would be to repeat the study with calorie intake held constant. Instead of this laborious exercise, a partial correlation analysis with calorie intake held artificially constant can be adequately performed, and would provide virtually the same result. Partial correlation analysis is performed using the SPSS module Correlations.

Command:

Analyze....Correlate....Partial....Variables: enter weight loss and calorie intake....Controlling for: enter exercise....OK.

Correlations

Control variables			Weightloss	Calorieintake
Exercise	Weightloss	Correlation	1.000	−0.548
		Significance (2-tailed)		0.000
		df	0	61
	Calorieintake	Correlation	−0.548	1.000
		Significance (2-tailed)	0.000	
		df	61	0

Correlations

Control variables			Weightloss	Exercise
Calorieintake	weightloss	Correlation	1.000	0.596
		Significance (2-tailed)		0.000
		df	0	61
	Exercise	Correlation	0.596	1.000
		Significance (2-tailed)	0.000	
		df	61	0

The upper table shows, that, with exercise held constant, calorie intake is a significant negative predictor of weight loss with a correlation coefficient of -0.548 and a p value of 0.0001. Also partial correlation with exercise as independent and calorie intake as controlling factor can be performed.

Command:

Analyze....Correlate....Partial....Variables: enter weight loss and exercise.... Controlling for: enter calorie intake....OK.

The lower table shows that, with calorie intake held constant, exercise is a significant positive predictor of weight loss with a correlation coefficient of 0.596 and a p-value of 0.0001.

Why do we no longer have to account interaction with partial correlations. This is simply because, if you hold a predictor fixed, this fixed predictor can no longer change and interact in a multiple regression model.

Also higher order partial correlation analyses are possible. E.g., age may affect all of the three variables already in the model. The effect of exercise on weight loss with calorie intake and age fixed can be assessed.

Command:

Analyze....Correlate....Partial....Variables: enter weight loss and exercise.... Controlling for: enter calorie intake and age....OK.

Correlations			Weightloss	Exercise
Control variables			Weightloss	Exercise
Age and calorieintake	Weightloss	Correlation	10.000	0.541
		Significance (2-talled)		0.000
		df	0	60
	Exercise	Correlation	0.541	1.000
		Significance (2-talled)	0.000	
		Df	60	0

In the above output sheet it can be observed that the correlation coefficient is still very significant.

Conclusion

Without the partial correlation approach the conclusion from this study would have been: no definitive conclusion about the effects of exercise and calorie intake is possible, because of a significant interaction between exercise and calorie intake. The partial correlation analysis allows to conclude that both exercise and calorie intake have a very significant linear relationship with weight loss effect.

Note

More background, theoretical and mathematical information of partial correlations methods is given in Machine Learning in Medicine Part One, Chap. 5, Partial correlations, pp 55–64, Springer Heidelberg Germany 2013.

Chapter 12
Canonical Regression for Overall Statistics of Multivariate Data (250 Patients)

General Purpose

To assess in datasets with multiple predictor and outcome variables, whether canonical analysis, unlike traditional multivariate analysis of variance (MANOVA), can provide overall statistics of combined effects.

Specific Scientific Question

The example of the Chaps. 7 and 8 is used once again. Twelve highly expressed genes are used to predict four measures of drug efficacy. We are more interested in the combined effect of the predictor variables on the outcome variables than we are in the separate effects of the different variables.

G1	G2	G3	G4	G16	G17	G18	G19	G24	G25	G26	G27	O1	O2	O3	O4
8	8	9	5	7	10	5	6	9	9	6	6	6	7	6	7
9	9	10	9	8	8	7	8	8	9	8	8	8	7	8	7
9	8	8	8	8	9	7	8	9	8	9	9	9	8	8	8
8	9	8	9	6	7	6	4	6	6	5	5	7	7	7	6
10	10	8	10	9	10	10	8	8	9	9	9	8	8	8	7
7	8	8	8	8	7	6	5	7	8	8	7	7	6	6	7
5	5	5	5	5	6	4	5	5	6	6	5	6	5	6	4
9	9	9	9	8	8	8	8	9	8	3	8	8	8	8	8
9	8	9	8	9	8	7	7	7	7	5	8	8	7	6	6
10	10	10	10	10	10	10	10	10	8	8	10	10	10	9	10
2	2	8	5	7	8	8	8	9	3	9	8	7	7	7	6
7	8	8	7	8	6	6	7	8	8	8	7	8	7	8	8
8	9	9	8	10	8	8	7	8	8	9	9	7	7	8	8

Var G1–27 = highly expressed genes estimated from their arrays' normalized ratios
Var O1–4 = drug efficacy scores (the variables 20–23 from the initial data file)

T. J. Cleophas and A. H. Zwinderman, *Machine Learning in Medicine - Cookbook*, 73
SpringerBriefs in Statistics, DOI: 10.1007/978-3-319-04181-0_12,
© The Author(s) 2014

The data from the first 13 patients are shown only (see extra.springer.com for the entire data file entitled "optscalingfactorplscanonical"). First, MANOVA (multivariate analysis of variance) was performed with the four drug efficacy scores as outcome variables and the twelve gene expression levels as covariates. We can now use SPSS 19.0. Start by opening the data file.

Canonical Regression

Command:
Click Analyze....click General Linear Model....click Multivariate....Dependent Variables: enter the four drug efficacy scores....Covariates: enter the 12 genes....OK.

	Effect value	F	Hypothesis df	Error df	p value
Intercept	0.043	2.657	4.0	234.0	0.034
Gene 1	0.006	0.362	4.0	234.0	0.835
Gene 2	0.27	1.595	4.0	234.0	0.176
Gene 3	0.042	2.584	4.0	234.0	0.038
Gene 4	0.013	0.744	4.0	234.0	0.563
Gene 16	0.109	7.192	4.0	234.0	0.0001
Gene 17	0.080	5.118	4.0	234.0	0.001
Gene 18	0.23	1.393	4.0	234.0	0.237
Gene 19	0.092	5.938	4.0	234.0	0.0001
Gene 24	0.045	2.745	4.0	234.0	0.029
Gene 25	0.017	1.037	4.0	234.0	0.389
Gene 26	0.027	1.602	4.0	234.0	0.174
Gene 27	0.045	2.751	4.0	234.0	0.029

The MANOVA table is given (F = F-value, df = degrees of freedom). It shows that MANOVA can be considered as another regression model with intercepts and regression coefficients. We can conclude that the genes 3, 16, 17, 19, 24, and 27 are significant predictors of all four drug efficacy outcome scores. Unlike ANOVA, MANOVA does not give overall p-values, but rather separate p-values for separate covariates. However, we are, particularly, interested in the combined effect of the set of predictors, otherwise called covariates, on the set of outcomes, rather than we are in modeling the separate variables. In order to asses the overall effect of the cluster of genes on the cluster of drug efficacy scores canonical regression is performed.

Command:
Click File....click New....click Syntax....the Syntax Editor dialog box is displayed....enter the following text: "manova" and subsequently enter all of the

outcome variables....enter the text "WITH"....then enter all of the gene-names
....then enter the following text:/discrim all alpha(1)/print = sig(eigen dim)....-
click Run.

Numbers variables (covariates v outcome variables)							
	Canon cor	Sq cor	Wilks L	F	Hypoth df	Error df	p
12 v 4	0.87252	0.7613	0.19968	9.7773	48.0	903.4	0.0001
7 v 4	0.87054	0.7578	0.21776	16.227	28.0	863.2	0.0001
7 v 3	0.87009	0.7571	0.22043	22.767	21.0	689.0	0.0001

The above table is given (cor = correlation coefficient, sq = squared, L = lambda, hypoth = hypothesis, df = degree of freedom, p = p-value, v = versus). The upper row, shows the result of the statistical analysis. The correlation coefficient between the 12 predictor and 4 outcome variables equals 0.87252. A squared correlation coefficient of 0.7613 means that 76 % of the variability in the outcome variables is explained by the 12 covariates. The cluster of predictors is a very significant predictor of the cluster of outcomes, and can be used for making predictions about individual patients with similar gene profiles. Repeated testing after the removal of separate variables gives an idea about relatively unimportant contributors as estimated by their coefficients, which are kind of canonical b-values (regression coefficients). The larger they are, the more important they are.

Canon Cor			
Model	12 v 4	7 v 4	7 v 3
Raw			
Outcome 1	−0.24620	−0.24603	0.25007
Outcome 2	−0.20355	−0.19683	0.20679
Outcome 3	−0.02113	−0.02532	
Outcome 4	−0.07993	−0.08448	0.09037
Gene 1		0.01177	
Gene 2		−0.01727	
Gene 3	−0.05964	−0.08344	0.08489
Gene 4		−0.02865	
Gene 16	−0.14094	−0.13883	0.13755
Gene 17	−0.12897	−0.14950	0.14845
Gene 18	−0.03276		
Gene 19	−0.10626	−0.11342	0.11296
Gene 24	−0.07148	−0.07024	0.07145
Gene 25	−0.00164		
Gene 26	−0.05443	−0.05326	0.05354
Gene 27	0.05589	0.04506	−0.04527

(continued)

(continued)

Canon Cor			
Model	12 v 4	7 v 4	7 v 3
Standardized			
Outcome 1	−0.49754	−0.49720	0.50535
Outcome 2	−0.40093	−0.38771	0.40731
Outcome 3	−0.03970	−0.04758	
Outcome 4	−0.15649	−0.16539	0.17693
Gene 1		0.02003	
Gene 2		−0.03211	
Gene 3	−0.10663	−0.14919	0.15179
Gene 4		−0.04363	
Gene 16	−0.30371	−0.29918	0.29642
Gene 17	−0.23337	−0.27053	0.26862
Gene 18	−0.06872		
Gene 19	−0.23696	−0.25294	0.25189
Gene 24	−0.18627	−0.18302	0.18618
Gene 25	−0.00335		
Gene 26	−0.14503	−0.14191	0.14267
Gene 27	0.12711	0.10248	−0.10229

The above table left column gives an overview of raw and standardized (z transformed) canonical coefficients, otherwise called canonical weights (the multiple b-values of canonical regression), (Canon Cor = canonical correlation coefficient, v = versus, Model = analysis model after removal of one or more variables). The outcome 3, and the genes 2, 4, 18 and 25 contributed little to the overall result. When restricting the model by removing the variables with canonical coefficients smaller than 0.05 or larger than −0.05 (the middle and right columns of the table), the results were largely unchanged. And so were the results of the overall tests (the 2nd and 3rd rows). Seven versus three variables produced virtually the same correlation coefficient but with much more power (lambda increased from 0.1997 to 0.2204, the F value from 9.7773 to 22.767, in spite of a considerable fall in the degrees of freedom. It, therefore, does make sense to try and remove the weaker variables from the model ultimately to be used. The weakest contributing covariates of the MANOVA were virtually identical to the weakest canonical predictors, suggesting that the two methods are closely related and one method confirms the results of the other.

Conclusion

Canonical analysis is wonderful, because it can handle many more variables than MANOVA, accounts for the relative importance of the separate variables and their interactions, provides overall statistics. Unlike other methods for combining the effects of multiple variables like factor analysis/partial least squares (Chap. 8), canonical analysis is scientifically entirely rigorous.

Note

More background, theoretical and mathematical information of canonical regression is given in Machine Learning in Medicine Part one, Chap. 8, Canonical regression, pp. 225–240, Springer Heidelberg Germany 2013.

Part III
Rules Models

Chapter 13
Neural Networks for Assessing Relationships that are Typically Nonlinear (90 Patients)

General Purpose

Unlike regression analysis which uses algebraic functions for data fitting, neural networks uses a stepwise method called the steepest decent method for the purpose. To asses whether typically nonlinear relationships can be adequately fit by this method.

Specific Scientific Question

Body surface is a better indicator for drug dosage than body weight. The relationship between body weight, length and surface are typically nonlinear. Can a neural network be trained to predict body surface of individual patients.

Var 1	Var 2	Var 3
30.50	138.50	10,072.90
15.00	101.00	6,189.00
2.50	51.50	1,906.20
30.00	141.00	10,290.60
40.50	154.00	13,221.60
27.00	136.00	9,654.50
15.00	106.00	6,768.20
15.00	103.00	6,194.10
13.50	96.00	5,830.20
36.00	150.00	11,759.00
12.00	92.00	5,299.40
2.50	51.00	2,094.50
19.00	121.00	7,490.80
28.00	130.50	9,521.70

Var 1 = weight (kg)
Var 2 = height (m)
Var 3 = body surface measured photometrically (cm^2)
The first 14 patients are shown only, the entire data file is entitled "neural networks" and is in extras.springer.com.

T. J. Cleophas and A. H. Zwinderman, *Machine Learning in Medicine - Cookbook*,   81
SpringerBriefs in Statistics, DOI: 10.1007/978-3-319-04181-0_13,
© The Author(s) 2014

The Computer Teaches Itself to Make Predictions

SPSS 19.0 is used for training and outcome prediction. It uses XML (eXtended Markup Language) files to store data. MLP stands for multilayer perceptron, and indicates the neural network methodology used. Start by opening the data file.

Command:
Click Transform....click Random Number Generators....click Set Starting Point....click Fixed Value (2000000)....click OK....click Analyze....Neural Networks.... Multilayer Perceptron....Dependent Variable: select body surface ....Factors: select weight and height....click Partitioning: set the training sample (7), test sample (3), hold out sample (0)....click Architecture: click Custom Architecture....set the numbers of hidden layers (2)....click Activation Function: click hyperbolic tangens....click Save: click Save predicted values or category for each dependent variable....click Export: click Export synaptic weight estimates to XML file....click Browse....File name: enter "exportnn"....click Save....Options: click Maximum training time Minutes (15)....click OK.

The output warns that in the testing sample some cases have been excluded from analysis because of values not occurring in the training sample. Minimizing the output sheets shows the data file with predicted values (MLP_PredictedValue).

They are pretty much similar to the measured body surface values. We will use linear regression to estimate the association between the two.

Command:
Analyze....Regresssion....Linear....Dependent: bodysurface   ....Independent: MLP_PredictedValue....OK.

The output sheets show that the r-value is 0.998, r-square 0.995, $p < 0.0001$. The saved XML file will now be used to compute the body surface in five individual patients.

Patient no	Weight	Height
1	36.00	130.50
2	28.00	150.00
3	12.00	121.00
4	19.00	92.00
5	2.50	51.00

Enter the above data in a new SPSS data file.

Command:
Utilities....click Scoring Wizard....click Browse....click Select....Folder: enter the exportnn.xml file....click Select....in Scoring Wizard click Next....click Use value substitution....click Next....click Finish.

The above data file now gives the body surfaces computed by the neural network with the help of the XML file.

Patient no	Weight	Height	Computed body surfaces
1	36.00	130.50	10,290.23
2	28.00	150.00	11,754.33
3	12.00	121.00	7,635.97
4	19.00	92.00	4,733.40
5	2.50	51.00	2,109.32

Conclusion

Multilayer perceptron neural networks can be readily trained to provide accurate body surface values of individual patients, and other nonlinear clinical outcomes.

Note

More background, theoretical and mathematical information of neural networks is available in Machine Learning Part One, Chaps. 12 and 13 entitled "Artificial intelligence, multilayer perceptron" and "Artificial intelligence, radial basis functions", pp. 145–156 and 157–166, Springer Heidelberg Germany 2013.

Chapter 14
Complex Samples Methodologies for Unbiased Sampling (9,678 Persons)

General Purpose

The research of entire populations is costly and obtaining information from selected samples instead is generally biased by selection bias. Complex sampling produces weighted, and, therefore, unbiased population estimates. This chapter is to assess whether this method can be trained for predicting health outcomes.

Specific Scientific Question

Can complex samples be trained to predict unbiased current health outcomes from previous health outcomes in individual members of an entire population.

Var 1	Var 2	Var 3	Var 4	Var 5	Var 6
1	1	1	9	19.26	3.00
1	1	1	7	21.11	6.00
1	1	1	9	22.42	9.00
1	1	1	7	20.13	12.00
1	1	1	5	16.37	15.00
1	1	1	8	20.49	18.00
1	1	1	7	20.79	21.00
1	1	1	7	17.52	24.00
1	1	1	7	18.12	27.00
1	1	1	6	18.60	30.00

Var 1 = neighborhood
Var 2 = town
Var 3 = county
Var 4 = time (years)
Var 5 = last health score
Var 6 = case identity number (defined as property ID)

T. J. Cleophas and A. H. Zwinderman, *Machine Learning in Medicine - Cookbook*,
SpringerBriefs in Statistics, DOI: 10.1007/978-3-319-04181-0_14,
© The Author(s) 2014

Prior health scores of a 9,768 member population recorded some 5–10 years ago were available as well as topographical information (the data file is entitled "complexsamples" and is in extras.springer.com. We wish to obtain information of individual current health scores. For that purpose the information of the entire data plus additional information on the current health scores from a random sample of 1,000 from this population were used. First, a *sampling plan* was designed with different counties, townships and neighborhoods weighted differently. A *random sample* of 1,000 was taken, and additional information was obtained from this random sample, and included.

The latter data file plus the *sampling plan* were, then, used for analysis. The SPSS modules complex samples (cs) "general linear model" and "ratios" modules were applied for analyses. A *sampling plan* of the above population data was designed using SPSS. Open in extras.springer.com the database entitled "complexsamples".

Command:

click Analyze....Complex Samples.... Select a sample.... click Design a sample, click Browse: select a map and enter a name, e.g., complexsamplesplan....click Next....Stratify by: select county....Clusters: select township....click Next...Type: Simple Random Sampling....click Without replacement....click Next....Units: enter Counts....click Value: enter 4....click Next....click Next....-click (Yes, add stage 2 now)....click Next...Stratify by: enter neighbourhood....next...Type: Simple   random   sampling....click   Without replacement....click Next....Units: enter proportions....click Value: enter 0.25....click Next....click Next....click (No, do not add another stage now)....-click Next...Do you want to draw a sample: click Yes....Click Custom value....enter 123....click Next....click External file, click Browse: select a map and enter a name, e.g., complexsamplessample ....click Save....click Next....click Finish.

In the original data file the weights of 1,006 randomly sampled individuals are now given. In the maps selected above we find two new files,

1. entitled "complexsamplesplan" (this map can not be opened, but it can in closed form be entered whenever needed during further complex samples analyses of these data), and
2. entitled "complexsamplessample" containing 1,006 randomly selected individuals from the main data file.

The latter data file is first completed with current health scores before the definitive analysis. Only of 974 individuals the current information could be obtained, and these data were added as a new variable (see "complexsamplessample" at extras.springer.com). Also "complexsamplesplan" has for convenience been made available at extras.springer.com.

The Computer Teaches Itself to Predict Current Health Scores from Previous Health Scores

We now use the above data files "complexsamplessample" and "complexsamplesplan" for predicting individual current health scores and odds ratios of current versus previous health scores. Also, an XML (eXtended Markup Language) file will be designed for analyzing future data. First, open "complexsamplessample".

Command:

Click Transform....click Random Number Generators....click Set Starting Point....click Fixed Value (2,000,000)....click OK....click Analyze....Complex Samples....General Linear Model....click Browse: select the appropriate map and enter complexsamplesplan....click Continue...Dependent variable: enter curhealthscore ....Covariates: enter last healthscores....click Statistics: mark Estimates, 95 % Confidence interval, t test....click Save....mark Predicted Values....in Export Model as XML click Browse....in appropriate folder enter File name: "exportcslin"....click Save....click Continue....click OK.

The underneath table gives the correlation coefficient and the 95 % confidence intervals. The lower part gives the data obtained through the usual commands [Analyze, Regression, Linear, Dependent (curhealthscore), Independent (s) (last healthscore), OK]. It is remarkable to observe the differences between the two analyses. The correlation coefficients are largely the same but their standard errors are respectively 0.158 and 0.044. The t value of the complex sampling analysis equals 5.315, while that of the traditional analysis equals no less than 19.635. Nonetheless, the reduced precision of the complex sampling analysis did not produce a statistically insignificant result, and, in addition, it was, of course, again adjusted for inappropriate probability estimates.

Parameter estimates[a]							
Parameter	Estimate	Std. error	95 % Confidence interval		Hypothesis test		
			Lower	Upper	t	df	Sig.
(Intercept)	8.151	2.262	3.222	13.079	3.603	12.000	0.004
lasthealthscore	0.838	0.158	0.494	1.182	5.315	12.000	0.000

[a] Model: curhealthscore = (Intercept) + lasthealthscore

Model		Coefficients[a]			t	Sig.
		Unstandardized coefficients		Standardized coefficients		
		B	Std. error	Beta		
1	(Constant)	7.353	0.677		10.856	0.000
	lasthealthscore	0.864	0.044	0.533	19.635	0.000

[a] Dependent variable: curhealthscore

The saved XML file will now be used to compute the predicted current health score in five individual patients from this population.

	Var 5
1	19.46
2	19.77
3	16.75
4	16.37
5	18.35

Var 5 = last health score

Enter the above data in a new SPSS data file.
Command:
Utilities....click Scoring Wizard....click Browse....click Select....Folder: enter the exportcslin.xml file....click Select....in Scoring Wizard click Next....mark Predicted Value....click Next....click Finish.
The above data file now gives the body surfaces computed by the neural network with the help of the XML file.

	Var 5	Var 6
1	19.46	24.46
2	19.77	24.72
3	16.75	22.19
4	16.37	21.87
5	18.35	23.53

Var 5 = last health score
Var 6 = predicted value of current health score

The Computer Teaches Itself to Predict Odds Ratios of Current Health Scores Versus Previous Health Scores

Open again the data file "complexsamplessample".

Command:
Click Transform....click Random Number Generators....click Set Starting Point.... click Fixed Value (2,000,000)....click OK....click Analyze....Complex Samples ....Ratios....click Browse: select the appropriate map and enter

"complexsamplesplan"....click Continue...Numerators: enter curhealthscore....
Denominator: enter last healthscore ....Subpopulations: enter County....click
Statistics: mark Standard error, Confidence interval (enter 95 %), Design
effect....click Continue....click OK.

The underneath table (upper part) gives the overall ratio and the ratios per
county plus 95 % confidence intervals. The design effects are the ratios of the
variances of the complex sampling method versus that of the traditional, otherwise
called simple random sampling (srs), method. In the given example the ratios are
mostly 3–4, which means that the uncertainty of the complex samples methodology is 3–4 times larger than that of the traditional method. However, this
reduction in precision is compensated for by the removal of biases due to the use
of inappropriate probabilities used in the srs method.

The lower part of the table gives the srs data obtained through the usual
commands [Analyze, Descriptive Statistics, Ratio, Numerator (curhealthscore),
Denominator (lasthealthscore), Group Variable (County), Statistics (means, confidence intervals etc.)]. Again the ratios of the complex samples and traditional
analyses are rather similar, but the confidence intervals are very different. E.g., the
95 % confidence intervals of the Northern County went from 1.172 to 1.914 in the
complex samples, and from 1.525 to 1.702 in the traditional analysis, and was thus
over 3 times wider.

Ratios 1

Numerator	Denominator	Ratio estimate	Standard error	95 % Confidence interval		Design effect
				Lower	Upper	
curhealthscore	lasthealthscore	1.371	0.059	1.244	1.499	17.566

Ratios 1

County	Numerator	Denominator	Ratio estimate	Standard error	95 % Confidence interval		Design effect
					Lower	Upper	
Eastern	curhealthscore	lasthealthscore	1.273	0.076	1.107	1.438	12.338
Southern	curhealthscore	lasthealthscore	1.391	0.100	1.174	1.608	21.895
Western	curhealthscore	lasthealthscore	1.278	0.039	1.194	1.362	1.518
Northern	curhealthscore	lasthealthscore	1.543	0.170	1.172	1.914	15.806

Ratio statistics for curhealthscore/lasthealthscore

Group	Mean	95 % Confidence interval for mean		Price related differential	Coefficient of dispersion	Coefficient of variation
		Lower bound	Upper bound			Median centered (%)
Eastern	1.282	1.241	1.323	1.007	0.184	24.3
Southern	1.436	1.380	1.492	1.031	0.266	33.4
Western	1.342	1.279	1.406	1.051	0.271	37.7
Northern	1.613	1.525	1.702	1.044	0.374	55.7
Overall	1.429	1.395	1.463	1.047	0.285	41.8

The confidence intervals are constructed by assuming a normal distribution for the ratios

In addition to the statistics given above, other complex samples statistics are possible, and they can be equally well executed in SPSS, that is if the data are appropriate. If you have a binary outcome variable (dichotomous) available, then logistic regression modeling is possible, if an ordinal outcome variable is available, complex samples ordinal regression, if time to event information is in the data, complex samples Cox regression can be performed.

Conclusion

Complex samples is a cost-efficient method for analyzing target populations that are large and heterogeneously distributed. Also it is time-efficient, and offers greater scope and deeper insight, because specialized equipments are feasible.

Traditional analysis of limited samples from heterogeneous target populations is a biased methodology, because each individual selected is given the same probability, and the spread in the data is, therefore, generally underestimated. In complex sampling this bias is adjusted for by assigning appropriate weights to each individual included.

Note

More background, theoretical and mathematical information of complex samples methodologies is given in Machine Learning in Medicine Part Three, Chap. 12, Complex samples, pp. 127–139, Springer Heidelberg Germany 2013.

Chapter 15
Correspondence Analysis for Identifying the Best of Multiple Treatments in Multiple Groups (217 Patients)

General Purpose

Multiple treatments for one condition are increasingly available, and a systematic assessment would serve optimal care. Research in this field to date is problematic. This chapter is to propose a novel method based on cross-tables, correspondence analysis.

Specific Scientific Question

Can correspondence analysis avoid the bias of multiple testing, and identify the best of multiple treatments in multiple groups.

Var 1	Var 2
1	1
1	1
1	1
1	1
1	1
1	1
1	1
1	1
1	1
1	1

(continued)

T. J. Cleophas and A. H. Zwinderman, *Machine Learning in Medicine - Cookbook*, SpringerBriefs in Statistics, DOI: 10.1007/978-3-319-04181-0_15, © The Author(s) 2014

(continued)

Var 1	Var 2
1	1
1	1

Var 1 = treatment modality (1–3)
Var 2 = response (1 = complete remission, 2 = partial
remission, 3 = no response)
Only the first 12 patients are given, the entire data file entitled
"correspondence analysis" is in extras.springer.com. 217
patients were randomly treated with one of three treatments
(treat = treatment) and produced one of three responses
(1 = complete remission, 2 = partial remission, 3 = no
response). We will use SPSS statistical software 19.0

Correspondence Analysis

First, a multiple groups Chi square test is performed. Start by opening the data file.

Command:
Analyze....Descriptive Statistics....Crosstabs....Row(s): enter treatment....
Column(s): enter remission, partial, no [Var 2]....click Statistics....mark Chi
square....click Continue....click Cell Display ....mark Observed....mark
Expected ....click Continue....OK.

Treatment* remission, partial, no crosstabulation

			Remission, partial, no			Total
			1.00	2.00	3.00	
Treatment	1.00	Count	19	21	18	58
		Expected count	21.6	10.7	25.7	58.0
	2.00	Count	41	9	39	89
		Expected count	33.2	16.4	39.4	89.0
	3.00	Count	21	10	39	70
		Expected count	26.1	12.9	31.0	70.0
Total		Count	81	40	96	217
		Expected count	81.0	40.0	96.0	217.0

The output file compares the observed counts (patients) per cell with the expected count, if no significant difference existed. Also, a Chi square value is given, 21.462 with 4° of freedom, p value < 0.0001. There is a significantly different pattern in numbers of responders between the different treatment groups. To find out what treatment is best a correspondence analysis is performed. For that purpose the individual Chi square values are calculated from the values of the above table according to the underneath equation.

$$\left[(\text{observed count} - \text{expected count})^2/\text{expected count}\right]$$

Then, the individual Chi square values are converted to similarity measures. With these values the software program creates a two-dimensional quantitative distance measure that is used to interpret the level of nearness between the treatment groups and response groups. We will use again SPSS 19.0 statistical software for the analysis.

Command:
Analyze....Dimension Reduction....Correspondence Analysis....Row: enter treatment....click Define Range....Minimum value: enter1....Maximum value: enter 3....click Update....Column: enter remission, partial, no [Var 2] ....click Define Range....Minimum value: enter1....Maximum value: enter 3....click Update....click Continue ....click Model....Distance Measure: click Chi square....click Continue....click Plots....mark Biplot....OK.

Remission				
Treatment		Yes	Partial	No
1	Residual	−2.6	10.3	−7.7
	$(o - e)^2/e$	0.31	9.91	2.31
	Similarity	−0.31	9.91	−2.31
2	Residual	7.9	−7.4	−0.4
	$(o - e)^2/e$	1.88	3.34	0.004
	Similarity	1.88	−3.34	−0.004
3	Residual	−4.1	−2.9	8.0
	$(o - e)^2/e$	0.64	0.65	2.65
	Similarity	−0.64	−0.65	2.65

The above table of similarity values is given in the output. Also the underneath plot of the coordinates of both the treatment groups and the response groups in a one two-dimensional plane is shown in the output. This plot is meaningful. As treatment group 2 and response group 1 tend to join, and treatment group 1 and response group 2 do, equally, so, we have reason to believe that treatment group 2 has the best treatment and treatment group 1 the second best. This is, because response group 1 has a complete remission, and response group 2 has a partial remission. If a 2 × 2 table of the treatment groups 1 and 2 versus the response groups 1 and 2 shows a significant difference between the treatments, then we can argue, that the best treatment is, indeed, significantly better than the second best treatment.

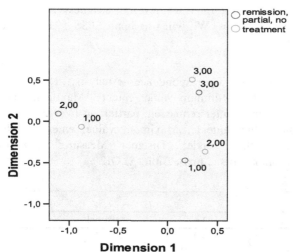

Dimension 1

For statistical testing response 1 and 2 versus treatment 1 and 2 recoding of the variables is required, but a simpler solution is to use a pocket calculator method for computing the Chi square value.

Response			
Treatment	1	2	Total
1	19	21	40
2	41	9	50
	60	30	90

$$\text{Chi} - \text{square} = \frac{[(9 \times 19) - (21 \times 41)]^2 \times 90}{60 \times 30 \times 50 \times 40}$$

$$= 11.9 \text{ with } 1° \text{ of freedom, } p < 0.0001$$

Treatment 2, indeed, produced significantly more complete remissions than did treatment 1, as compared to the partial remissions.

Conclusion

In our example correspondence analysis was able to demonstrate which one of three treatments was best, and it needed, instead of *multiple* 2×2 tables, only a single 2×2 table for that purpose. The advantage of this procedure will be even more obvious, if larger sets of categorical data have to be assessed. A nine cells data file would require only nine 2×2 tables to be tested, a sixteen cells data file would require thirty-six of them. This procedure will almost certainly produce significant effects by chance rather than true effects, and is, therefore, rather meaningless. In contrast, very few tests are needed, when a correspondence analysis is used to identify the proximities in the data, and the risk of type I errors is virtually negligible.

Note

We should add that, instead of a two-dimensional analysis as used in the current chapter, correspondence analysis can also be applied for multidimensional analyses. More background, theoretical and mathematical information of correspondence analysis is given in Machine Learning in Medicine Part Two, Chap. 13, Correspondence analysis, pp. 129–137, Springer Heidelberg Germany 2013.

Chapter 16
Decision Trees for Decision Analysis (1,004 and 953 Patients)

General Purpose

Decision trees are, so-called, non-metric or non-algorithmic methods adequate for fitting nominal and interval data. This chapter is to assess whether decision trees can be appropriately applied to predict health risks and improvements.

Specific Scientific Question

Can decision trees be trained to predict in individual future patients risk of infarction and ldl (low density lipoprotein) cholesterol decrease.

Decision Trees with a Binary Outcome

Var 1	Var 2	Var 3	Var 4	Var 5	Var 6
0.00	44.86	1.00	0.00	1.00	2.00
0.00	42.71	2.00	0.00	1.00	2.00
0.00	43.34	3.00	0.00	2.00	2.00
0.00	44.02	3.00	0.00	1.00	2.00
0.00	67.97	1.00	0.00	2.00	2.00
0.00	40.31	2.00	0.00	2.00	2.00
0.00	66.56	1.00	0.00	2.00	2.00
0.00	45.95	1.00	0.00	2.00	2.00
0.00	52.27	1.00	0.00	1.00	2.00
0.00	43.86	1.00	0.00	1.00	2.00
0.00	46.58	3.00	0.00	2.00	1.00

Var 1 = infarct_rating (0.00 no, 1.00 yes)
Var 2 = age (years)
Var 3 = cholesterol_level (1.00–3.00)
Var 4 = smoking (0.00 no, 1.00 yes)
Var 5 = education (levels 1.00 and 2.00)
Var 6 = weight_level (levels 1.00 and 2.00)

T. J. Cleophas and A. H. Zwinderman, *Machine Learning in Medicine - Cookbook*, SpringerBriefs in Statistics, DOI: 10.1007/978-3-319-04181-0_16, © The Author(s) 2014

The data from the first 13 patients are shown only. See extra.springer.com for the entire data file entitled "decisiontreebinary": in a 1,004 patient data file of risk factors for myocardial infarct a so-called Chi squared automatic interaction (CHAID) model is used for analysis. Also an XML (eXtended Markup Language) will be exported for the analysis of future data. Start by opening the data file.

Command:
Click Transform....click Random Number Generators....click Set Starting Point.... click Fixed Value (2000000)....click OK....click Classify....Tree....Dependent Variable: enter infarct rating....Independent Variables: enter age, cholesterol level, smoking, education, weight level....Growing Method: select CHAID....click Categories: Target mark yes....Continue....click Output: mark Tree in table format....Criteria: Parent Node type 200, Child Node type 100....click Continue.... click Save: mark Terminal node number, Predicted probabilities.... in Export Tree Model as XML mark Training sample....click Browse........in File name enter "exportdecisiontreebinary" ....in Look in: enter the appropriate map in your computer for storage....click Save....click OK.

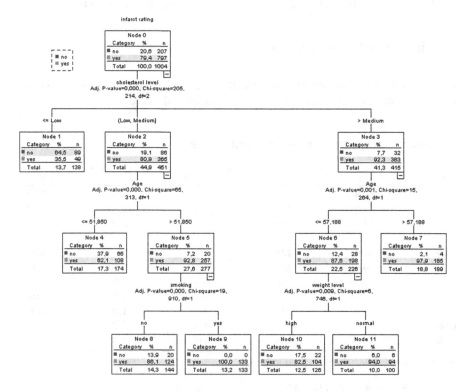

The output sheets show the decision tree and various tables. The Cholesterol level is the best predictor of the infarct rating. For low cholesterol the cholesterol level is the only significant predictor of infarction: only 35.5 % will have an infarction. In the medium and high cholesterol groups age is the next best predictor. In the elderly with medium cholesterol smoking contributes considerably to the risk of infarction. In contrast, in the younger with high cholesterol those with normal weight are slightly more at risk of infarction than those with high weights. For each node (subgroup) the number of cases, the Chi square value, and level of significance is given. A p value <0.05 indicates that the difference between the 2×2 or 3×2 tables of the paired nodes are significantly different from one another. All of the p-values were very significant.

The risk and classification tables indicate that the category infarction predicted by the model is wrong in $0.166 = 16.6 \%$ of the cases (underneath table). A correct prediction of 83.4% is fine. However, in those without an infarction no infarction is predicted in only 43.0% of the cases (underneath table).

Risk	
Estimate	Std. error
0.166	0.012

Growing method: CHAID
Dependent variable: infarct rating

Classification			
Observed	Predicted		
	No	Yes	Percent correct (%)
No	89	118	43.0
Yes	49	748	93.9
Overall percentage (%)	13.7	86.3	83.4

Growing method: CHAID
Dependent variable: infarct rating

When returning to the original data file we will observe 3 new variables, (1) the terminal node number, (2) the predicted probabilities of no infarction for each case, (3) the predicted probabilities of yes infarction for each case. In a binary logistic regression it can be tested that the later variables are much better predictors of the probability of infarction than each of the original variables are. The saved XML file will now be used to compute the predicted PAF rate in 6 novel patients with the following characteristics. For convenience the XML file is given in extras.springer.com.

Var 2	Var 3	Var 4	Var 5	Var 6
59.16	2.00	0.00	1.00	2.00
53.42	1.00	0.00	2.00	2.00
43.02	2.00	0.00	2.00	2.00
76.91	3.00	1.00	1.00	1.00
70.53	2.00	0.00	1.00	2.00
47.02	3.00	1.00	1.00	1.00

Var 2 = age (years)
Var 3 = cholesterol_level (1.00–3.00)
Var 4 = smoking (0.00 no, 1.00 yes)
Var 5 = education (level 1.00 and 2.00)
Var 6 = weight_level (1.00 and 2.00)

Enter the above data in a new SPSS data file.

Command:
Utilities....click Scoring Wizard....click Browse....click Select....Folder: enter the exportdecisiontreebinary.xml file....click Select....in Scoring Wizard click Next....mark Node Number....mark Probability of Predicted Category....click Next....click Finish.

The above data file now gives the individual predicted nodes numbers and probabilities of infarct for the six novel patients as computed by the linear model with the help of the XML file. Enter the above data in a new SPSS data file.

Var 2	Var 3	Var 4	Var 5	Var 6	Var 7	Var 8
59.16	2.00	0.00	1.00	2.00	8.00	0.86
53.42	1.00	0.00	2.00	2.00	1.00	0.64
43.02	2.00	0.00	2.00	2.00	4.00	0.62
76.91	3.00	1.00	1.00	1.00	7.00	0.98
70.53	2.00	0.00	1.00	2.00	8.00	0.86
47.02	3.00	1.00	1.00	1.00	11.00	0.94

Var 2 = age
Var 3 = cholesterol_level
Var 4 = smoking
Var 5 = education
Var 6 = weight_level
Var 7 = predicted node number
Var 8 = predicted probability of infarct

Decision Trees with a Continuous Outcome

Var 1	Var 2	Var 3	Var 4	Var 5	Var 6
3.41	0	1	3.00	3	0
1.86	−1	1	2.00	3	1
0.85	−2	1	1.00	4	1
1.63	−1	1	2.00	3	1
6.84	4	0	4.00	2	0
1.00	−2	0	1.00	3	0
1.14	−2	1	1.00	3	1
2.97	0	1	3.00	4	0
1.05	−2	1	1.00	4	1
0.63	−2	0	1.00	3	0
1.18	−2	0	1.00	2	0
0.96	−2	1	1.00	2	0
8.28	5	0	4.00	2	1

Var 1 = ldl_reduction
Var 2 = weight_reduction
Var 3 = gender
Var 4 = sport
Var 5 = treatment_level
Var 6 = diet

For the decision tree with continuous outcome the classification and regression tree (CRT) model is applied. A 953 patient data file is used of various predictors of ldl (low-density-lipoprotein)-cholesterol reduction including weight reduction, gender, sport, treatment level, diet. The file is in extras.springer.com and is entitled "decisiontreecontinuous". The file is opened.

Command:
Click Transform....click Random Number Generators....click Set Starting Point.... click Fixed Value (2000000)....click OK....click Analyze....Classify...Tree.... Dependent Variable: enter ldl_reduction.... Independent Variables: enter weight reduction, gender, sport, treatment level, diet....Growing Methods: select CRT ....click Criteria: enter Parent Node 300, Child Node 100....click Output: Tree mark Tree in table format....click Continue....click Save....mark Terminal node number....mark Predicted value....in Export Tree Model as XML mark Training sample....click Browse........in File name enter "exportdecision-treecontinuous" ....,in Look in: enter the appropriate map in your computer for storage....click Save....click OK.

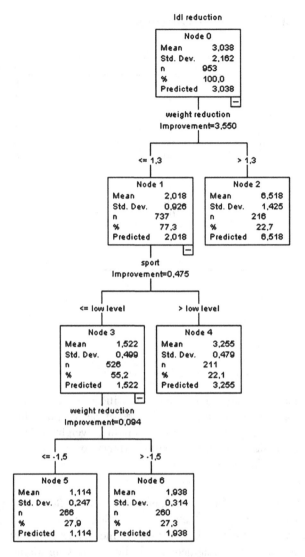

The output sheets show the classification tree. Only weight reduction and sport significantly contributed to the model, with the overall mean and standard deviation dependent variable ldl cholesterol in the parent (root) node. Weight reduction with a cut-off level of 1.3 units is the best predictor of ldl reduction. In the little weight reduction group sport is the best predictor. In the low sport level subgroup again weight reduction is a predictor, but here there is a large difference between weight gain (<−1.5 units) and weight loss (>−1.5 units). Minimizing the output shows the original data file. It now contains two novel variables, the npde classification and the predicted value of ldl cholesterol reduction. They are entitled NodeId and PredictedValue. The saved XML (eXtended Markup Language) file will now be used to compute the predicted node classification and value of ldl cholesterol reduction in 5 novel patients with the following characteristics. For convenience the XML file is given in extras.springer.com.

Var 2	Var 3	Var 4	Var 5	Var 6
−0.63	1.00	2.00	1.00	0.00
2.10	0.00	4.00	4.00	1.00
−1.16	1.00	2.00	1.00	1.00
4.22	0.00	4.00	1.00	0.00
−0.59	0.00	3.00	4.00	1.00

Var 2 = weight_reduction
Var 3 = gender
Var 4 = sport
Var 5 = treatment_level
Var 6 = diet

Enter the above data in a new SPSS data file.

Command:
Utilities....click Scoring Wizard....click Browse....click Select....Folder: enter the exportdecisiontreecontinuous.xml file....click Select....in Scoring Wizard click Next....mark Node Number....mark Predicted Value....click Next....click Finish.

The above data file now gives individually predicted node classifications and predicted ldl cholesterol reductions as computed by the linear model with the help of the XML file.

Var 2	Var 3	Var 4	Var 5	Var 6	Var 7	Var 8
−0.63	1.00	2.00	1.00	0.00	6.00	1.94
2.10	0.00	4.00	4.00	1.00	2.00	6.52
−1.16	1.00	2.00	1.00	1.00	6.00	1.94
4.22	0.00	4.00	1.00	0.00	2.00	6.52
−0.59	0.00	3.00	4.00	1.00	4.00	3.25

Var 2 = weight_reduction
Var 3 = gender
Var 4 = sport
Var 5 = treatment_level
Var 6 = diet
Var 7 = predicted node classification
Var 8 = predicted ldl cholesterol reduction

Conclusion

The module decision trees can be readily trained to predict in individual future patients risk of infarction and ldl (low density lipoprotein) cholesterol decrease. Instead of trained XML files for predicting about future patients, also syntax files are possible for the purpose. They perform better if predictions from multiple instead of single future patients are requested.

Note

More background, theoretical and mathematical information of decision trees as well as the steps for utilizing syntax files is available in Machine Learning in Medicine Part Three, Chap. 14, entitled "Decision trees", pp. 153–168, Springer Heidelberg, Germany 2013.

Chapter 17
Multidimensional Scaling for Visualizing Experienced Drug Efficacies (14 Pain-Killers and 42 Patients)

General Purpose

To individual patients, objective criteria of drug efficacy, like pharmaco-dynamic/kinetic and safety measures may not mean too much, and patients' personal opinions are important too. This chapter is to assess whether multidimensional scaling can visualize subgroup differences in experienced drug efficacies, and whether data-based dimensions can be used to match dimensions as expected from pharmacological properties.

Specific Scientific Question

Can proximity and preference scores of pain-killers as judged by patient samples be used for obtaining insight in the real priorities both in populations and in individual patients. Can the data-based dimensions as obtained by this procedure be used to match dimensions as expected from pharmacological properties.

Proximity Scaling

	Var 1	Var 2	Var 3	Var 4	Var 5	Var 6	Var 7	Var 8	Var 9	Var 10	Var 11	Var 12	Var 13	Var 14
1	0													
2	8	0												
3	7	2	0											
4	5	4	5	0										
5	8	5	4	6	0									
6	7	5	6	6	8	0								

(continued)

T. J. Cleophas and A. H. Zwinderman, *Machine Learning in Medicine - Cookbook*, SpringerBriefs in Statistics, DOI: 10.1007/978-3-319-04181-0_17, © The Author(s) 2014

(continued)

	Var 1	Var 2	Var 3	Var 4	Var 5	Var 6	Var 7	Var 8	Var 9	Var 10	Var 11	Var 12	Var 13	Var 14
7	4	5	6	3	7	4	0							
8	8	5	4	6	3	8	7	0						
9	3	7	9	4	8	7	5	8	0					
10	5	6	7	6	9	4	4	9	6	0				
11	9	5	4	6	3	8	7	3	8	9	0			
12	9	4	3	7	5	7	7	5	8	9	5	0		
13	4	6	6	3	7	5	4	8	4	5	7	7	0	
14	6	6	7	6	8	2	4	9	7	3	9	7	5	0

Var 1–14 one by one distance scores of the pain-killers 1–14, mean estimates of 20 patients (scale 0–10). The 14 pain-killers are also given in the first column. The data file is entitled "proxscal" and is in extras.springer.com

The above matrix mean scores can be considered as one by one distances between all of the medicines connected with one another by straight lines in 14 different ways. Along an x- and y-axis they are subsequently modeled using the equation: the distance between drug i and drug j $= \sqrt{[(x_i - x_j)^2 + (y_i - y_j)^2]}$. SPSS statistical software 19.0 will be used for analysis. Start by opening the data file.

Command:
Analyze....Scale....Multidimensional scaling (PROXSCAL)....Data Format: click The data are proximities....Number of Sources: click One matrix source....One Source: click The proximities are in a matrix across columns....click Define.... enter all variables (medicines) into "Proximities"....Model: Shape: click Lower-triangular matrix....Proximity Transformation: click Interval....Dimensions: Minimum: enter 2....Maximum: enter 2....click Continue....click Plots....mark Common space....mark Transformed proximities versus distances....click Continue ....click: Output....mark Common space coordinates....mark Multiple stress measures....click Continue....click OK.

Stress and fit measures	
Normalized raw stress	0.00819
Stress-I	0.09051[a]
Stress-II	0.21640[a]
S-Stress	0.02301[b]
Dispersion accounted for (D.A.F.)	0.99181
Tucker's coefficient of congruence	0.99590

PROXSCAL minimizes normalized raw stress
[a] Optimal scaling factor = 1.008
[b] Optimal scaling factor = 0.995

The output sheets gives the uncertainty of the model (stress = standard error) and dispersion values. The model is assumed to appropriately describe the data if they are respectively <0.20 and approximately 1.0.

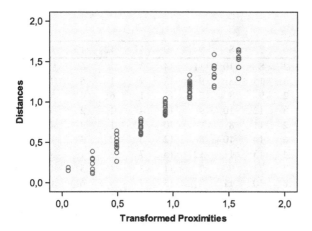

Also, a plot of the actual distances as observed versus the distances fitted by the statistical program is given. A perfect fit should produce a straight line, a poor fit produces a lot of spread around a line or even no line at all. The figure is not perfect but it shows a very good fit as expected from the stress and fit measures.

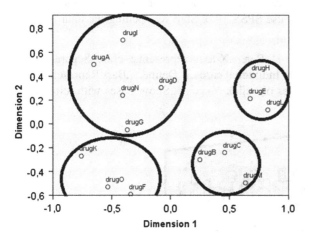

Finally, the above figure shows the most important part of the outcome. The standardized x- and y-axes values give some insight in the relative position of the medicines according to perception of our study population. Four clusters are identified. Using Microsoft's drawing commands we can encircle the clusters as identified. The cluster at the upper right quadrant comprises high priorities of the patients along both the x- and the y-axis. The cluster at the lower left quadrant comprises low priorities of the patients along both axes. If, pharmacologically, the drugs in the right upper quadrant were highly potent with little side effects, then the patients' priorities would fairly match the pharmacological properties of the medicines.

Preference Scaling

Var 1	2	3	4	5	6	7	8	9	10	11	12	13	14	15
12	13	7	4	5	2	8	10	11	14	3	1	6	9	15
14	11	6	3	10	4	15	8	9	12	7	1	5	2	13
13	10	12	14	3	2	9	8	7	11	1	6	4	5	15
7	14	11	3	6	8	12	10	9	15	4	1	2	5	13
14	9	6	15	13	2	11	8	7	10	12	1	3	4	5
9	11	15	4	7	6	14	10	8	12	5	2	3	1	13
9	14	5	6	8	4	13	11	12	15	7	2	1	3	10
15	10	12	6	8	2	13	9	7	11	3	1	5	4	14
13	12	2	4	5	8	10	11	3	15	7	9	6	1	14
15	13	10	7	6	4	9	11	12	14	5	2	8	1	3
9	2	4	13	8	5	1	10	6	7	11	15	14	12	3

Var 1–15 preference scores (1 = most preferred, 15 = least preferred)
Only the first 11 patients are given. The entire data file is entitled "prefscal" and is in
extras.springer.com

To 42 patients 15 different pain-killers are administered, and the patients are
requested to rank them in order of preference from 1 "most preferred" to 15 "least
preferred". First will try and draw a three dimensional view of the individually
assigned preferences. We will use SPSS 19.0. Start by opening the data file.

Command:
Graphs....Legacy Dialogs....3-D Bar....X-axis represents: click Separate variables....Z-axis represents: click Individual cases....Define....Bars Represent: enter
pain-killers 1–15....Show Cases on: click Y-axis....Show Cases with: click Case
number....click OK.

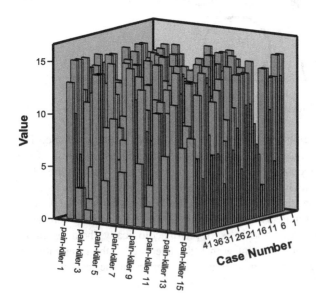

The above figure shows the result: a very irregular pattern consisting of multiple areas with either high or low preference is observed. We will now perform a preference scaling analysis. Like with proximity scaling, preference assessments is mapped in a 2 dimensional plane with the rank orders of the medicines as measures of distance between the medicines. Two types of maps are constructed: an aggregate map giving average distances of the entire population or individual maps of single patients, and an ideal point map where ideal points have to be interpreted as a map with ideal medicines, one for each patient. SPSS 19.0 is used once more.

Command:
Analyze....Scale....Multidimensional Unfolding (PREFSCAL)....enter all variables (medicines) into "Proximities"....click Model....click Dissimilarities.... Dimensions: Minimum enter 2 ....Maximum enter 2....Proximity Transformations: click Ordinal ....click Within each row separately....click Continue....click Options: imputation by: enter Spearman....click Continue....click Plots: mark Final common space....click Continue....click Output: mark Fit measures ....mark Final common space....click Continue....click OK.

Measures		
Iterations		115
Final function value		0.7104127
Function value parts	Stress part	0.2563298
	Penalty part	1.9688939
Badness of fit	Normalized stress	0.0651568
	Kruskal's stress-I	0.2552582
	Kmskal's stress-ll	0.6430926
	Young's S-stress-I	0.3653360
	Young's S-stress-ll	0.5405226
Goodness of fit	Dispersion accounted for	0.9348432
	Variance accounted for	0.7375011
	Recovered preference orders	0.7804989
	Spearman's rho	0.8109694
	Kendall's tau-b	0.6816390
Variation coefficients	Variation proximities	0.5690984
	Variation transformed proximities	0.5995274
	Variation distances	0.4674236
Degeneracy indices	Sum-of-squares of DeSarbo's intermixedness indices	0.2677061
	Shepard's rough nondegeneracy index	0.7859410

The above table gives the stress (standard error) and fit measures. The best fit distances as estimated by the model are adequate: measures of stress including normalized stress and Kruskal's stress-I are close to 0.20 or less, the value of dispersion measures (Dispersion Accounted For) is close to 1.0. The table also shows whether there is a risk of a *degenerate* solution, otherwise called loss function. The individual proximities have a tendency to form circles, and when averaged for obtaining average proximities, there is a tendency for the average treatment places to center in the middle of the map. The solution is a penalty term, but in our example we need not worry. The DeSarbo's and Shepard criteria are close to respectively 0 and 80 %, and no penalty adjustment is required.

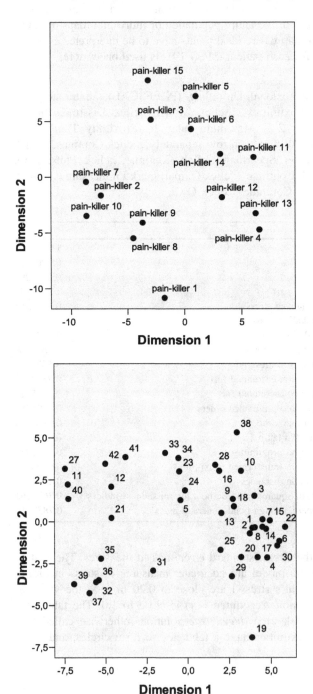

The above figure (upper graph) gives the most important part of the output. The standardized x- and y-axes values of the upper graph give some insight in the relative position of the medicines according to our study population. The results can be understood as the relative position of the medicines according to the perception of our study population. Both the horizontal and the vertical dimension appears to discriminate between different preferences. The lower graph gives the patients' *ideal points*. The patients seem to be split into two clusters with different preferences, although with much variation along the y-axis. The dense cluster in the right lower quadrant represented patients with preferences both along the x- and y-axis. Instead of two-dimensions, multidimensional scaling enables to assess multiple dimensions each of which can be assigned to one particular cause for proximity. This may sound speculative, but if the pharmacological properties of the drugs match the place of the medicines in a particular dimension, then we will be more convinced that the multi-dimensional display gives, indeed, an important insight in the real priorities of the patients. In order to address this issue, we will now perform a multidimensional scaling procedure of the above data including three dimensions.

Command:
Analyze....Scale....Multidimensional Unfolding (PREFSCAL)....enter all variables (medicines) into "Proximities"....click Model....click Dissimilarities.... Dimensions: Minimum enter 3 ....Maximum enter 3....Proximity Transformations: click Ordinal ....click Within each row separately....click Continue....click Options: imputation by: enter Spearman....click Continue....click Plots: mark Final common space....click Continue....click Output: mark Fit measures ....mark Final common space....click Continue....click OK.

Final column coordinates

Pain-killer no.	Dimension		
	1	2	3
1	−2.49	−9.08	−4.55
2	−7.08	−1.81	1.43
3	−3.46	3.46	−2.81
4	5.41	−4.24	1.67
5	−0.36	6.21	5.25
6	0.17	1.88	−3.27
7	−7.80	−2.07	−1.59
8	−5.17	−4.18	2.91
9	4.75	−0.59	4.33
10	−6.80	−4.83	0.27
11	6.22	2.50	0.88
12	3.71	−1.27	−0.49
13	5.30	−2.95	1.51
14	2.82	1.66	−2.09
15	−4.35	2.76	−6.72

The output sheets shows the standardized mean preference values of the different pain-killers as x-, y-, and z-axis coordinates. The best fit outcome of the three-dimensional (3-D) model can be visualized in a 3-D figure. SPSS 19.0 is used. First cut and paste the data from the above table to the preference scaling file or another file. Then proceed.

Command:
Graphs....Legacy Dialogs....Scatter/Dot....click 3-D Scatter....click Define....
Y-Axis: enter dimension 1....X-Axis: enter dimension 2....Z-Axis: enter dimension 3....click OK.

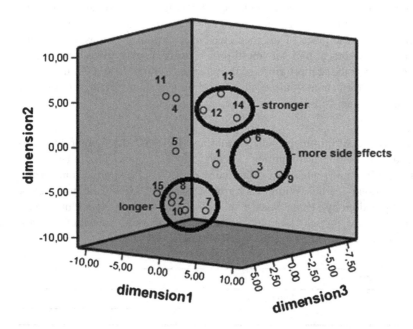

The above figure gives the best fit outcome of a 3-dimensional scaling model. Three clusters were identified, consistent with patients' preferences along an x-, y-, and z-axis. Using Microsoft's drawing commands we can encircle the clusters as identified. In the figure an example is given of how pharmacological properties could be used to explain the cluster pattern.

Conclusion

Multidimensional scaling is helpful both to underscore the pharmacological properties of the medicines under studies, and to identify what effects are really important to patients, and uses for these purposes estimated proximities as surrogates for counted estimates of patients' opinions. Multidimensional scaling can, like regression analysis, be used two ways, (1) for estimating preferences of treatment modalities in a population, (2) for assessing the preferred treatment modalities in individual patients.

Note

More background, theoretical and mathematical information of multidimensional scaling is given in Machine Learning in Medicine Part Two, Chap. 12, Multidimensional scaling, pp. 115–127, Springer Heidelberg Germany 2013.

•

Chapter 18
Stochastic Processes for Long Term Predictions from Short Term Observations

General Purpose

Markov modeling, otherwise called stochastic processes, assumes that per time unit the same % of a population will have an event, and it is used for long term predictions from short term observations. This chapter is to assess whether the method can be applied by non-mathematicians using an online matrix-calculator.

Specific Scientific Questions

If per time unit the same % of patients will have an event like surgery, medical treatment, a complication like a co-morbidity or death, what will be the average time before such events take place.

Example 1 Patients with three states of treatment for a disease are checked every 4 months. The underneath matrix is a so-called transition matrix. The states 1–3 indicate the chances of treatment: $1 =$ no treatment, $2 =$ surgery, $3 =$ medicine. If you are in state 1 today, there will be a $0.3 = 30$ % chance that you will receive no treatment in the next 4 months, a $0.2 = 20$ % chance of surgery, and a $0.5 = 50$ % chance of medicine treatment. If you are still in state 1 (no treatment) after 4 months, there will again be a 0.3 chance that this will be the same in the second 4 month period etc. So, after 5 periods the chance of being in state 1 equals $0.3 \times 0.3 \times 0.3 \times 0.3 \times 0.3 = 0.00243$. The chance that you will be in the states 2 or 3 is much larger, and there is something special about these states. Once you are in these states you will never leave them anymore, because the patients who were treated with either surgery or medicine are no longer followed in this study. That this happens can be observed from the matrix: if you are in state 2, you will have a chance of $1 = 100$ % to stay in state 2 and a chance of $0 = 0$ % not to do so. The same is true for the state 3.

T. J. Cleophas and A. H. Zwinderman, *Machine Learning in Medicine - Cookbook*, SpringerBriefs in Statistics, DOI: 10.1007/978-3-319-04181-0_18, © The Author(s) 2014

State in current time	State in next period (4 months)		
	1	2	3
1	0.3	0.2	0.5
2	0	1	0
3	0	0	1

Now we will compute what will happen with the chances of a patient in the state 1 after several 4 month periods.

4 month period	Chances of being in state:		
	State 1	State 2	State 3
1st	30 %	20 %	50 %
2nd	$30 \times 0.3 = 9$ %	$20 + 0.3 \times 20 = 26$ %	$50 + 0.3 \times 50 = 65$ %
3rd	$9 \times 0.3 = 3$ %	$26 + 9 \times 0.2 = 27.8$ %	$65 + 9 \times 0.5 = 69.5$ %
4th	$3 \times 0.3 = 0.9$ %	$27.8 + 3 \times 0.2 = 28.4$ %	$69.5 + 3 \times 0.5 = 71.0$ %
5th	$0.9 \times 0.3 = 0.27$ %	$28.4 + 0.9 \times 0.2 = 28.6$ %	$71.0 + 0.9 \times 0.5 = 71.5$ %

Obviously, the chances of being in the states 2 or 3 will increase, though increasingly slowly, and the chance of being in state 1 is, ultimately, going to approximate zero. In clinical terms: postponing the treatment does not make much sense, because everyone in the no treatment group will eventually receive a treatment and the ultimate chances of surgery and medicine treatment are approximately 29 and 71 %. With larger matrices this method for calculating the ultimate chances is rather laborious. Matrix algebra offers a rapid method.

State in current time	State in next period (4 months)		
	1	2	3
1	$[0.3]$	$[0.2 \quad 0.5]$	Matrix Q	Matrix R
2	$[0]$	$[1 \quad 0]$	Matrix O	Matrix I
3	$[0]$	$[0 \quad 1]$		

The states are called transient, if they can change (the state 1), and absorbing if not (the states 2 and 3). The original matrix is partitioned into four submatrices, otherwise called the canonical form:

[0.3]	Upper left corner
	This square matrix Q can be sometimes very large with rows and columns respectively presenting the transient states
[0.2 0.5]	Upper right corner
	This R matrix presents in rows the chance of being absorbed from the transient state
$\begin{bmatrix} 1 & 0 \end{bmatrix}$	Lower right corner
$\begin{bmatrix} 0 & 1 \end{bmatrix}$	This identity matrix I presents rows and columns with chances of being in the absorbing states, the I matrix must be adjusted to the size of the Q matrix (here it will look like [1] instead of $\begin{bmatrix} 1 & 0 \end{bmatrix}$
	$\begin{bmatrix} 0 & 1 \end{bmatrix}$
[0]	Lower left corner
[0]	This is a matrix of zeros (0 matrix)

From the above matrices a fundamental matrix (F) is constructed.

$$[(\text{matrix I}) - (\text{matrix R})]^{-1} = [0.7]^{-1} = 10/7$$

With larger matrices a matrix calculator, like the Bluebit Online Matrix Calculator can be used to compute the matrix to the -1 power by clicking "Inverse".

The fundamental matrix F equals 10/7. It can be interpreted as the average time, before someone goes into the absorbing state ($10/7 \times 4$ months $= 5.714$ months). The product of the fundamental matrix F and the R matrix gives more exact chances of a person in state 1 ending up in the states 2 and 3.

$$F \times R = (10/7) \times [0.2 \quad 0.5] = [2/7 \quad 5/7] = [0.285714 \quad 0.714286].$$

The two latter values add up to 1.00, which indicates a combined chance of ending up in an absorbing state equal to 100 %.

Example 2 Patients with three states of treatment for a chronic disease are checked every 4 months.

State in current time	State in next period (4 months)		
	1	2	3
1	0.3	0.6	0.1
2	0.45	0.5	0.05
3	0	0	1

The above matrix of three states and second periods of time gives again the chances of different treatment for a particular disease, but it is slightly different from the first example. Here state 1 = no treatment state, state 2 = medicine treatment, state 3 = surgery state. We assume that medicine can be stopped while surgery is irretrievable, and, thus, an absorbing state. We first partition the matrix.

State in current time	State in next period (4 months)		
	1	2	3
1	$\begin{bmatrix} 0.3 & 0.6 \end{bmatrix}$	$[0.1]$	Matrix Q Matrix R
2	$\begin{bmatrix} 0.45 & 0.5 \end{bmatrix}$	$[0.05]$	
3	$\begin{bmatrix} 0 & 0 \end{bmatrix}$	$[1]$	Matrix O Matrix I

The R matrix} $\begin{bmatrix} 0.1 \\ 0.05 \end{bmatrix}$ is in the upper right corner.

The Q matrix $\begin{bmatrix} 0.3 & 0.6 \\ 0.45 & 0.5 \end{bmatrix}$ is in the left upper corner.

The I matrix $[1]$ is in the lower right corner, and must be adjusted, before it

can be subtracted from the Q matrix according to $\begin{bmatrix} 1 & 0 \\ 0 & 1 \end{bmatrix}$

The 0 matrix $[0\ 0]$ is in the lower left corner.

$$I - Q = \begin{bmatrix} 1 & 0 \\ 0 & 1 \end{bmatrix} - \begin{bmatrix} 0.3 & 0.6 \\ 0.45 & 0.5 \end{bmatrix} = \begin{bmatrix} 0.7 & 0.6 \\ 0.45 & 0.5 \end{bmatrix}$$

The inverse of $[I - Q]$ is obtained by marking "Inverse" at the online Bluebit Matrix Calculator and equals

$$[I - Q] = \begin{bmatrix} 6.25 & 7.5 \\ 5.625 & 8.75 \end{bmatrix} = \text{fundamental matrix F.}$$

It is interpreted as the average periods of time before some transient state goes into the absorbing state:
$(6.25 + 7.5 = 13.75) \times 4$ months for the patients in state 1 first and state 2 s,
$(5.625 + 8.75 = 14.375) \times 4$ months for the patients in state 2 first and state 1 s).
Finally, the product of matrix F times matrix R is calculated. It gives the chances of ending up in the absorbing state for those starting in the states 1 and 2.

$$\begin{bmatrix} 6.25 & 7.5 \\ 5.625 & 8.75 \end{bmatrix} \times \begin{bmatrix} 0.1 \\ 0.05 \end{bmatrix} = \begin{bmatrix} 1.00 \\ 1.00 \end{bmatrix}$$

Obviously the chance of both the transient states for ending up in the absorbing state is $1.00 = 100\ \%$.

Example 3 State 1 = stable coronary artery disease (CAD),
  state 2 = complications,
  state 3 = recovery state,
  state 4 = death state).

State in current time	State in next period (4 months)			
	1	2	3	4
1	0.95	0.04	0	0.01
2	0	0	0.9	0.1
3	0	0.3	0.3	0.4
4	0	0	0	1

If you take higher powers of this transition matrix (P), you will observe long-term trends of this model. For that purpose use the matrix calculator and square the transition matrix (P^2 gives the chances in the 2nd 4 month period etc.) and compute also higher powers (P^3, P^4, P^5, etc.).

$$P^2$$
$$\begin{matrix} 0.903 & 0.038 & 0.036 & 0.024 \\ 0.000 & 0.270 & 0.270 & 0.460 \\ 0.000 & 0.090 & 0.360 & 0.550 \\ 0.000 & 0.000 & 0.000 & 1.000 \end{matrix}$$

$$P^6$$
$$\begin{matrix} 0.698 & 0.048 & 0.063 & 0.191 \\ 0.000 & 0.026 & 0.064 & 0.910 \\ 0.000 & 0.021 & 0.047 & 0.931 \\ 0.000 & 0.000 & 0.000 & 1.000 \end{matrix}$$

The above higher order transition matrices suggest that with rising powers, and, thus, after multiple 4 month periods, there is a general trend towards the absorbing state: in each row the state 4 value continually rises. In the end we all will die, but in order to be more specific about the time, a special matrix like the one described in the previous examples is required. In order to calculate the precise time before the transient states go into the absorbing state, we need to partition the initial transition matrix.

State in current time	State in next period (4 months)			
	1	2	3	4
1	$\begin{bmatrix} 0.95 & 0.04 & 0 \\ 0 & 0 & 0.9 \\ 0 & 0.3 & 0.3 \end{bmatrix}$	$\begin{bmatrix} 0.01 \\ 0.1 \\ 0.4 \end{bmatrix}$	Matrix Q	Matrix R
2				
3				
4	$\begin{bmatrix} 0 & 0 & 0 \end{bmatrix}$	$[1]$	Matrix O	Matrix I

$$F = (I - Q)^{-1}$$

$$I - Q = \begin{bmatrix} 1 & 0 & 0 \\ 0 & 1 & 0 \\ 0 & 0 & 1 \end{bmatrix} - \begin{bmatrix} 0.95 & 0.04 & 0.0 \\ 0.0 & 0.0 & 0.9 \\ 0.0 & 0.3 & 0.3 \end{bmatrix}$$

$$F = \begin{bmatrix} 0.05 & -0.04 & 0 \\ 0.0 & 1.0 & -0.9 \\ 0.0 & -0.3 & 0.7 \end{bmatrix}^{-1}$$

The online Bluebit Matrix calculator (mark inverse) produces the underneath result.

$$F = \begin{bmatrix} 20.0 & 1.302 & 1.674 \\ 0.0 & 1.628 & 2.093 \\ 0.0 & 0.698 & 2.326 \end{bmatrix}$$

The average time before various transient states turn into the absorbing state (dying in this example) is given.

State 1 : $(20 + 1.302 + 1.674) \times 4$ months $= 91.904$ months
State 2 : $(0.0 + 1.628 + 2.093) \times 4$ months $= 14.884$ months
State 3 : $(0.0 + 0.698 + 2.326) \times 4$ months $= 12.098$ months

The chance of dying for each state is computed from matrix F times matrix R (click multiplication, enter the data in the appropriate fields and click calculate.

$$F.R = \begin{bmatrix} 20.0 & 1.302 & 1.674 \\ 0.0 & 1.628 & 2.093 \\ 0.0 & 0.698 & 2.326 \end{bmatrix} \times \begin{bmatrix} 0.01 \\ 0.1 \\ 0.4 \end{bmatrix} = \begin{bmatrix} 1.0 \\ 1.0 \\ 1.0 \end{bmatrix}$$

Like in the previous examples again the products of the matrices F and R show that all of the states end up with death. However, in the state 1 this takes more time than it does in the other states.

Conclusion

Markov chains are used to analyze the long-term risks of reversible and irreversible complications including death. The future is not shown, but it is shown, what will happen, if everything remains the same. Markov chains assume, that the chance of an event is not independent, but depends on events in the past.

Note

More background, theoretical and mathematical information of Markov chains (stochastic modeling) is given in Machine Learning in Medicine Part Three, Chaps. 17 and 18, "Stochastic processes: stationary Markov chains" and "Stochastic processes: absorbing Markov chains", pp 195–204 and 205–216, Springer Heidelberg Germany 2013.

Chapter 19
Optimal Binning for Finding High Risk Cut-offs (1445 Families)

General Purpose

Optimal binning is a so-called non-metric method for describing a continuous predictor variable in the form of best fit categories for making predictions. Like binary partitioning (Machine Learning in Medicine Part One, Chap. 7, Binary partitioning, pp. 79–86, Springer Heidelberg, Germany, 2013) it uses an exact test called the entropy method, which is based on log likelihoods. It may, therefore, produce better statistics than traditional tests. In addition, unnecessary noise due to continuous scaling is deleted, and categories for identifying patients at high risk of particular outcomes can be identified. This chapter is to assess its efficiency in medical research.

Specific Scientific Question

Increasingly unhealthy lifestyles cause increasingly high risks of overweight children. We are, particularly, interested in the best fit cut-off values of unhealthy lifestyle estimators to maximize the difference between low and high risk.

Var 1	Var 2	Var 3	.	Var 4	Var 5
0	11	1		8	0
0	7	1		9	0
1	25	7		0	1
0	11	4		5	0
1	5	1		8	1
0	10	2		8	0

(continued)

T. J. Cleophas and A. H. Zwinderman, *Machine Learning in Medicine - Cookbook*, SpringerBriefs in Statistics, DOI: 10.1007/978-3-319-04181-0_19, © The Author(s) 2014

(continued)

Var 1	Var 2	Var 3	Var 4	Var 5
0	11	1	6	0
0	7	1	8	0
0	7	0	9	0
0	15	3	0	0

Var 1 = fruitvegetables (0 = no, 1 = yes)
Var 2 = unhealthysnacks (times per week)
Var 3 = fastfoodmeal (times per week)
Var 4 = physicalactivities (times per week)
Var 5 = overweightchildren (0 = no, 1 = yes)

Only the first 10 families are given, the entire data file is entitled "optimalbinning" and is in extras.springer.com.

Optimal Binning

SPSS 19.0 is used for analysis. Start by opening the data file.

Command:
Transform….Optimal Binning….Variables into Bins: enter fruitvegetables, unhealthysnacks, fastfoodmeal, physicalactivities….Optimize Bins with Respect to: enter "overweightchildren"….click Output….Display: mark Endpoints….mark Descriptive statistics….mark Model Entropy….click Save: mark Create variables that contain binned data….click OK.

Descriptive statistics					
	N	Minimum	Maximum	Number of distinct values	Number of bins
Fruitvegetables/week	1,445	0	34	33	2
Unhealthysnacks/week	1,445	0	42	1,050	3
Fastfoodmeal/week	1,445	0	21	1,445	2
Physicalactivities/week	1,445	0	10	1,385	2

In the output the above table is given. N = the number of adults in the analysis, Minimum/Maximum = the range of the original continuous variables, Number of Distinct Values = the separate values of the continuous variables as used in the binning process, Number of Bins = the number of bins (= categories) generated and is smaller than the initials separate values of the same variables.

Model entropy	
	Model entropy
Fruitvegetables/week	0.790
Unhealthysnacks/week	0.720
Fastfoodmeal/week	0.786
Physicalactivities/week	0.805

Smaller model entropy Indicates higher predictive accuracy of the binned variable on guide variable overweight children

Model Entropy gives estimates of the usefulness of the bin models as predictor models for probability of overweight: the smaller the entropy, the better the model. Values under 0.820 indicate adequate usefulness.

Fruitvegtables\week

Bin	End point		Number of cases by level of overweight children		
	Lower	Upper	No	Yes	Total
1	a	14	802	340	1,142
2	14	a	274	29	303
Total			1,076	369	1,445

Unhealthysnacks/week

Bin	End point		Number of cases by level of overweight children		
	Lower	Upper	No	Yes	Total
1	a	12	830	143	973
2	12	19	188	126	314
3	19	a	58	100	158
Total			1,076	369	1,445

Fastfood meal/week

Bin	End point		Number of cases by level of overweight children		
	Lower	Upper	No	Yes	Total
1	a	2	896	229	1,125
2	2	a	180	140	320
Total			1,076	369	1,445

Physicalactivities/week

Bin	End point		Number of cases by level of overweight children		
	Lower	Upper	No	Yes	Total
1	a	8	469 ·	221	690
2	8	a	607	148	755
Total			1,076	369	1,445

Each bin is computed as Lower ≤ physicalactivities/week < Upper
[a] Unbounded

The above tables show the high risk cut-offs for overweight children of the four predicting factors. E.g., in 1,142 adults scoring under 14 units of fruit/vegetable per week, are put into bin 1 and 303 scoring over 14 units per week, are put into bin 2. The proportion of overweight children in bin 1 is much larger than it is in bin 2: $340/1,142 = 0.298$ (30 %) and $29/303 = 0.096$ (10 %). Similarly high risk cut-offs are found for

unhealthy snacks less than 12, 12–19, and over 19 per week
fastfood meals less than 2, and over 2 per week
physical activities less than 8 and over 8 per week.

These cut-offs can be used as meaningful recommendation limits to future families.
When we return to the dataview page, we will observe that the four variables have been added in the form of bin variables (with suffix _bin). They can be used as outcome variables for making predictions from other variables like personal characteristics of parents. Also they can be used, instead of the original variable, as predictors in regression modeling. A binary logistic regression with overweight children as dependent variable will be performed to assess their predictive strength as compared to that of the original variables. SPSS 19.0 will again be used.

Command:
Analyze....Regression....Binary Logistic....Dependent: enter overweight children ....Covariates: enter fruitvegetables, unhealthysnack, fastfoodmeal, physicalactivities....click OK.

Variables in the equation

		B	S.E.	Wald	df	Sig.	Exp(B)
Step 1[a]	Fruitvegetables	−0.092	0.012	58.775	1	0.000	0.912
	Unhealthysnacks	0.161	0.014	127.319	1	0.000	1.175
	Fastfoodmeal	0.194	0.041	22.632	1	0.000	1.214
	Physicalactivities	0.199	0.041	23.361	1	0.000	1.221
	Constant	−4.008	0.446	80.734	1	0.000	0.018

[a] Variable(s) entered on step 1: fruitvegetables, unhealthysnacks, fastfoodmeal, physicalactivities

The output shows that the predictors are very significant independent predictors of overweight children. Next the bin variable will be used.

Command:

Analyze....Regression....Binary Logistic....Dependent: enter overweight children ....Covariates: enter fruitvegetables_bin, unhealthysnack_bin, fastfoodmeal_bin, physicalactivities_bin....click OK.

Variables in the equation							
		B	S.E.	Wald	df	Sig.	Exp(B)
Step1[a]	Fruitvegetables_bin	−1.694	0.228	55.240	1	0.000	0.184
	Unhealth ys nacks_bin	1.264	0.118	113.886	1	0.000	3.540
	Fastfoodmeal_bin	0.530	0.169	9.827	1	0.002	1.698
	Physicalactivities_bin	0.294	0.167	3.086	1	0.079	1.341
	Constant	−2.176	0.489	19.803	1	0.000	0.114

[a] Variable(s) entered on step 1: fruitvegetables_bin, unhealthysnacks_bin, fastfoodmeal_bin, physicalactivities_bin

If $p < 0.10$ is used to indicate statistical significance, all of the bin variables are independent predictors, though at a somewhat lower level of significance than the original variables. Obviously, in the current example some precision is lost by the binning procedure. This is, because information may be lost if you replace a continuous variable with a binary or nominal one. Nonetheless, the method is precious for identifying high risk cut-offs for recommendation purposes.

Conclusion

Optimal binning variables instead of the original continuous variables may either produce (1) better statistics, because unnecessary noise due to the continuous scaling may be deleted (2) worse statistics, because information may be lost if your replace a continuous variable with a binary one. It is more adequate than traditional analyses, if categories are considered clinically more relevant

Note

More background, theoretical and mathematical information of optimal binning is given in Machine Learning in Medicine Part Three, Chap. 5, Optimal binning, pp. 37–48, Springer Heidelberg Germany 2013.

Chapter 20
Conjoint Analysis for Determining the Most Appreciated Properties of Medicines to be Developed (15 Physicians)

General Purpose

Products like articles of use, food products, or medicines have multiple characteristics. Each characteristic can be measured in several levels, and too many combinations are possible for a single person to distinguish. Conjoint analysis models a limited, but representative and meaningful subset of combinations, which can, subsequently, be presented to persons for preference scaling. The chapter is to assess whether this method is efficient for the development of new medicines.

Specific Scientific Question

Can conjoint analysis be helpful to pharmaceutical institutions for determining the most appreciated properties of medicines they will develop.

Constructing an Analysis Plan

A novel medicine is judged by 5 characteristics:

1. safety expressed in 3 levels,
2. efficacy in 3,
3. price in 3,
4. pill size in 2,
5. prolonged activity in 2 levels.

From the levels $3 \times 3 \times 3 \times 2 \times 2 = 108$ combinations can be formed, which is too large a number for physicians to distinguish. In addition, some combinations, e.g., high price and low efficacy will never be prefered and could be

T. J. Cleophas and A. H. Zwinderman, *Machine Learning in Medicine - Cookbook*, 129
SpringerBriefs in Statistics, DOI: 10.1007/978-3-319-04181-0_20,
© The Author(s) 2014

skipped from the listing. Instead, a limited but representative number of profiles is selected. SPSS statistical software 19.0 is used for the purpose.

Command:
Data....Orthogonal Design....Generate....Factor Name: enter safety....Factor Label: enter safety design....click Add....click ?....click Define Values: enter 1, 2, 3 on the left, and A, B, C on the right side....Do the same for all of the characteristics (here called factors)....click Create a new dataset....Dataset name: enter medicine_plan....click Options: Minimum number of cases: enter 18....mark Number of holdout cases: enter 4....Continue....OK.

The output sheets show a listing of 22, instead of 108, combinations with two new variables (status_ and card_) added. The variable Status_ gives a "0" to the first 18 combinations used for subsequent analyses, and "1" to holdout combinations to be used by the computer for checking the validity of the program. The variable Card_ gives identification numbers to each combination. For further use of the model designed so far, we will first need to perform the Display Design commands.

Command:
Data....Orthogonal Design....Display....Factors: transfer all of the characteristics to this window....click Listing for experimenter....click OK.

The output sheet now shows a plan card, which looks virtually identical to the above 22 profile listing. It must be saved. We will use the name medicine_plan for the file. For convenience the design file is given on the internet at extras.springer.com. The next thing is to use SPSS' syntax program to complete the preparation for real data analysis.

Command:
click File....move to Open....move to Syntax....enter the following text....
   CONJOINT PLAN = 'g:medicine_plan.sav'
   /DATA = 'g:medicine_prefs.sav'
   /SEQUENCE = PREF1 TO PREF22
   /SUBJECT = ID
   /FACTORS = SAFETY EFFICACY (DISCRETE)
   PRICE (LINEAR LESS)
   PILLSIZE PROLONGEDACTIVITY (LINEAR MORE)
   /PRINT = SUMMARYONLY.

Save this syntax file at the directory of your choice. Note: the conjoint file entitled "conjoint" only works, if both the plan file and the data file to be analyzed are correctly entered in the above text. In our example we saved both files at a USB stick (recognised by our computer under the directory "g:"). For convenience the conjoint file entitled "conjoint" is also given at extras.springer.com. Prior to use it should also be saved at the USB-stick.

The 22 combinations including the 4 holdouts, can now be used to perform a conjoint analysis with real data. For that purpose 15 physicians are requested to express their preferences of the 22 different combinations.

The preference scores are entered in the data file with the IDs of the physicians as a separate variable in addition to the 22 combinations (the columns). For convenience the data file entitled "medicine_prefs" is given at extras.springer.com, but, if you want to use it, it should first be saved at the USB stick. The conjoint analysis can now be successfully performed.

Performing the Final Analysis

Command:

Open the USB stick....click conjoint....the above syntax text is shown....click Run...select All.

Model description		
	No. of levels	Relation to ranks or scores
Safety	3	Linear (more)
Efficacy	3	Linear (more)
Price	3	Linear (less)
Pillsize	2	Discrete
Prolongedactivity	2	Discrete

All factors are orthogonal

The above table gives an overview of the different characteristics (here called factors), and their levels used to construct an analysis plan of the data from our data file.

Utilities			
		Utility estimate	Std. error
Pillsize	Large	−1.250	0.426
	Small	1.250	0.426
Prolongedactivity	No	−0.733	0.426
	Yes	0.733	0.426
Safety	A	1.283	0.491
	B	2.567	0.983
	C	3.850	1.474
Efficacy	High	−0.178	0.491
	Medium	−0.356	0.983
	Low	−0.533	1.474
Price	$4	−1.189	0.491
	$6	−2.378	0.983
	$8	−3.567	1.474
(Constant)		10.328	1.761

The above table gives the utility scores, which are the overall levels of the preferences expressed by the physicians. The meaning of the levels are given:

safety level C: best safety
efficacy level high: best efficacy
pill size 2: smallest pill
prolonged activity 2: prolonged activity present
price $8: most expensive pill.

Generally, higher scores mean greater preference. There is an inverse relationship between pill size and preference, and between pill costs and preference. The safest pill and the most efficaceous pill were given the best preferences.

However, the regression coefficients for efficacy were, statistically, not very significant. Nonetheless, they were included in the overall analysis by the software program. As the utility estimates are simply linear regression coefficients, they can be used to compute total utilities (add-up preference scores) for a medicine with known characteristic levels. An interesting thing about the methodology is that, like with linear regression modeling, the characteristic levels can be used to calculate an individual add-up utility score (preference score) for a pill with e.g., the underneath characteristics:

(1) pill size (small) + (2) prolonged activity (yes) + safety (C) + efficacy (high) + price   ($4) = 1.250 + 0.733 + 3.850 − 0.178 − 1.189 + constant (10.328) = 14.974.

For the underneath pill the add-up utility score is, as expected, considerably lower.

(1) pill size (large) + (2) prolonged activity (no) + safety (A) + efficacy (low) + price   ($8) = − 1.250 − 0.733 + 1.283 − 0.533 − 3.567 + constant (10.328) = 5.528.

The above procedure is the real power of conjoint analysis. It enables to predict preferences for combinations that were not rated by the physicians. In this way you will obtain an idea about the preference to be received by a medicine with known characteristics.

Importance values	
Pillsize	15.675
Prolongedactivity	12.541
Safety	28.338
Efficacy	12.852
Price	30.594

Averaged importance score

The range of the utility (preference) scores for each characteristic is an indi-cation of how important the characteristic is. Characteristics with greater ranges play a larger role than the others. As observed the safety and price are the most important preference producing characteristics, while prolonged activity, efficacy, and pill size appear to play a minor role according to the physicians' judgments. The ranges are computed such that they add-up to 100 (%).

Coefficients	
	B coefficient Estimate
Safety	1.283
Efficacy	−0.178
Price	−1.189

The above table gives the linear regression coefficients for the factors that are specified as linear. The interpretation of the utility (preference) score for the cheapest pill equals $4 \times (-1.189) = -4.756$

Correlations[a]	Value	Sig.
Pearson's R	0.819	0.000
Kendall's tau	0.643	0.000
Kendall's tau for holdouts	0.333	0.248

[a] Correlations between observed and estimated preferences

The correlation coefficients between the observed preferences and the prefer-ences calculated from conjoint model shows that the correlations by Pearson and Kendall's method are pretty good, indicating that the conjoint methodology pro-duced a sensitive prediction model. The regression analysis of the holdout cases is intended as a validity check, and produced a pretty large p value of 24.8 %. Still it means that we have about 75 % to find no type I error in this procedure.

Number of reversals			
Factor	Efficacy		9
	Price		5
	Safety		4
	Prolongedactivity		0
	Pillsize		0
Subject	1	Subject 1	1
	2	Subject 2	0
	3	Subject 3	0
	4	Subject 4	1
	5	Subject 5	3
	6	Subject 6	1
	7	Subject 7	3
	8	Subject 8	2
	9	Subject 9	1
	10	Subject 10	0
	11	Subject 11	1
	12	Subject 12	1
	13	Subject 13	0
	14	Subject 14	1
	15	Subject 15	3

Finally, the conjoint program reports the physicians (here the subjects) whose preference was different from what was expected. Particularly in the efficacy characteristic there were 9 of the 15 physicians who chose differently from expected, underlining the limited role of this characteristic.

Conclusion

Conjoint analysis is helpful to pharmaceutical institutions for determining the most appreciated properties of medicines they will develop. Disadvantage include: (1) it is pretty complex; (2) it may be hard to respondents to express preferences; (3) other characteristics not selected may be important too, e.g., physical and pharmacological factors.

Note

More background, theoretical and mathematical information of conjoint modeling is given in Machine Learning in Medicine Part Three, Chap. 19, Conjoint analysis, pp. 217–230, Springer Heidelberg Germany 2013.

Index

T. J. Cleophas and A. H. Zwinderman, *Machine Learning in Medicine - Cookbook*,   135
SpringerBriefs in Statistics, DOI: 10.1007/978-3-319-04181-0,
© The Author(s) 2014